Big Living
by ANGELA SANDLER

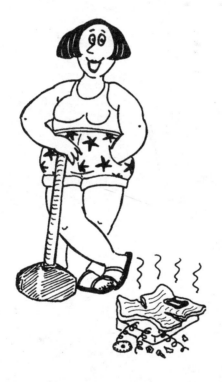

metro

First published in Great Britain in 1997
by Metro Books (an imprint of Metro Publishing Limited),
19 Gerrard Street, London W1V 7LA

British Library Cataloguing in Publication Data. A CIP record of this
book is available on request from the British Library.

ISBN 1 900512 16 5

10 9 8 7 6 5 4 3 2 1

Illustrations by Richard Burgess

Cartoons © Viv Quillin
*More space to put things, Sledgehammer and scales, Big bums are back in,
Easier to spot in a crowd* were first published in *Yes!* magazine

Typeset by Sally Brock, High Wycombe, Buckinghamshire.
Printed in Great Britain by Clays Ltd, St. Ives plc

Big Living

THIS BOOK IS AIMED AT ALL WOMEN

WHO ARE A SIZE 16 PLUS

AND ARE PUTTING THEIR LIFE ON HOLD

UNTIL THEY ARE A SIZE 16 MINUS

ACKNOWLEDGEMENTS

For their encouragement, comments and input: Judy Barnett, Deri Ben Atar, Lynn Greenfield, Yvonne Greensite AMFIC, Caroline Osborne, Suzi Pickles AMFIC (Director of the Colour Company), Sylvia Rose, Mary Evans Young for pointing me in the right direction with my opening chapters, Cheryl Lanyon for her patient editing and getting to grips with my subject so thoroughly.

David, my husband, for encouraging and believing in me and always being there when I need him.

Contents

Introduction

*A*re you a size 16 plus who hates to look in the mirror? Or are you a large woman, perfectly happy with your shape but longing to know how to make the best of your looks? In this book I draw on my own experience of being large, as well as my expertise as an image consultant, to show how you can accept your looks, improve your image and feel at ease with friends, family and at work. I'll pass on tips that will help you to *enjoy* being yourself; to look in the mirror and *like* what you see. I want to share with you the secret of being large, looking good and feeling great.

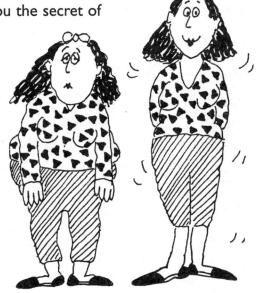

Learn to feel good about yourself and spot the difference!

Other books have been written on this subject — but few by someone like me, a large woman who has faced the struggle and emerged successfully on the other side.

When you feel good about yourself, it shows in everything you do. You succeed far more — in your appearance and achievements — than you would ever have believed possible, simply by having confidence.

Do you ever wear clothes that are too small because you don't feel you deserve anything new until you're slim? Have you given up on make-up because you feel a mess and it just isn't worth bothering? Be honest, have you ever thought, *'I'll do it when I'm slim'*?

In my career as an image consultant, I've come across these attitudes time and time again. Many larger women haven't been shown how to look good when they are a size 16 plus, so they won't treat themselves to anything until they are at least a size 16 minus. They don't look their best and their self-esteem suffers — though large women often blame this directly on their size and inability to diet, rather than on the fact that they're not making the best of themselves.

I have been guilty of all of these things.

I'll make an effort when I've just lost a stone or two, I suspect some of you are thinking. But look at it this way: dieting is a downward spiral. When you're on a diet, you feel miserable because you deprive yourself of one of your favourite things — *food*. Despite your good intentions, you dwell on what you're missing, feel resentful, and perhaps succumb to a treat 'just once'. Then you feel guilty about your lack of willpower as well as your size and your self-image takes a further downward plunge. You're caught in the diet trap.

A Controversial Idea

If you recognise that you are in the diet trap I've just described, I'd like to suggest a controversial approach. Instead of filling this book with dieting tips, I have concentrated on practical suggestions to make you feel comfortable with the size you are and love what is there now. If, later, you happen to lose weight, then have your clothes taken in while you gradually build up a new wardrobe of smaller sizes. But, meanwhile, learn how to look good today. If you are dieting successfully, that's wonderful, but I would still advise you to buy clothes that fit *now,* that you look good in *now.* If finances are tight, have large clothes taken in so that you look and feel good in everything you wear.

Flattery Gets You Everywhere

When you dress in styles, fabrics and colours that flatter you, you look good and feel better about yourself, no matter what the tape measure or scales say. And when you feel good, you're more likely to be able to stop dieting and learn to feel happy about your body. Just by wearing something which flatters your shape and colouring you can visually lose up to one stone in weight without the scales budging a fraction. I'm going to show you how you can dress in this way, without following rigid rules or having to throw your whole wardrobe out and start again.

Once you're looking your best at your present size, you can decide whether you really do want to torture yourself by dieting, or whether to make the most of your assets and stay as you are. Believe me, there is no reason why you shouldn't be large and look good. Here's how the revelation began for me.

Fourteen years ago, long before I had any intention of taking a course in 'Image, Colour and Style', I decided I needed advice on how to look good and went to see an image consultant.

It was just before my fortieth birthday. My wardrobe was a riot of colours and styles, I was uncertain with my make-up, and although sometimes I felt I'd got it all together and was complementing my looks, at other times I could see it just wasn't right. And I cared!

When I went to see the image consultant, I found myself in a class of eight women — all sizes 8–14. I certainly learned a lot about the right colours to wear and the make-up to complement them, but the consultant, a slip of a size 10, didn't let me forget my 24/26 size for one minute! She kept telling me which styles would suit me *when I had lost some weight*. She said I'd look good in floaty chiffon for the evening… 'but not at the moment, darling — you'd look like a ship in full sail'. The class laughed. Though I managed a polite grin, I was not amused.

That session was a turning-point for me. It took me three years to come to terms with my size (the size I still am today), and gradually to replace the clothes which weren't doing me any favours with new, flattering ones. Many of my clients manage to do it in less than six months. Others take longer than I did. It isn't a race and it doesn't matter how long it takes you. *But if you don't begin, you'll never get there.*

During those three years I started to use my experiences to help friends, small and large, organise their wardrobes, before deciding to do this professionally.

The first company I approached for training as an image consultant told me to come back when I was slimmer, as my size projected the 'wrong image'. I'm still not sure where I found the courage to approach another company, and I thank Barbara Jacques of the Academy of Colour and Style from the bottom of my heart for training me and not allowing my size to be an issue. I now train image consultants for The Colour Company and, ironically, am far more successful than the svelte trainer who turned me down ten years ago.

Real Life Encouragement

There are many real-life stories of large women in this book. Some have put their life on hold for years because of their weight, others have never let their weight stand in the way of their progress. I hope the tales will entertain and inspire you: if you are young and large, to get to grips with this subject now. If you are not so young, the advice is the same — it's never too late.

I hope this book will persuade you to:

- **Come to terms with your weight**
- **Stop dieting**
- **Sort out your wardrobe and start afresh (without breaking the bank).**
- **Wear colours and styles that suit and flatter you**

CHAPTER ONE

Living for Today

'DON'T PUT YOUR LIFE ON HOLD'

'DRESS FOR WHAT YOU ARE — NOT WHAT YOU WOULD LIKE TO BE'

In my work, I give presentations to many groups: secretaries' clubs; charity organisations; women's groups; senior corporate staff; women returning to work, amongst others. Whatever the audience, my first question is always, 'Do you have a wardrobe full of clothes and nothing to wear?' It inevitably raises a groan. Every woman, regardless of her shape, size or weight, ruefully admits that it is true.

But for the larger members of the audience it hits an even more tender spot. Not only do these women have a wardrobe full of clothes and nothing to wear, they often have a spare wardrobe full of clothes one or two sizes too small for them — and sometimes a suitcase full of yet more clothes that are even smaller. Those of you who get up every morning, look in the wardrobe and see lots of clothes that are too small, then look at yourself in the mirror and see someone who is too big to fit into them — do you have any idea what you are doing to yourself?

Let's be realistic. If you are large (and I'm talking about carrying excess weight, not just being naturally big-boned) then, unless you have a medical condition, it may be because, like me, you love food and can't, or don't want to, diet. Or there may be psychological factors that make you overeat.

Some experts believe there are genetic reasons for being large and this may be why some of you who have lost weight on a diet find it hard to stay slim (although other experts feel that genes are responsible in only a very few instances). According to those who see a genetic link, every time you lose weight your body is 'programmed' to go back to its genetically-set former level, so you have to keep on dieting to maintain weight loss. If you are genetically predisposed to be a certain weight (in other words, if you are naturally a big-boned size 16, for example), you are trying to achieve the impossible by constantly dieting. If you love food, you can't sustain this unequal battle. If food is a joy to you, dieting is going to make you miserable.

Food is not like cigarettes — you can't just give it up. The words 'going on a diet' mean that at some point you will come *off* it; but every time you do, you feel guilty and feed your brain with bad messages about your willpower and worth.

Have you ever considered *not* dieting? You're large, you like your food, you would like to look and feel good. Wouldn't it be easier to do this if you stayed the same size and really worked at achieving the look good/feel good factor at your natural, comfortable weight?

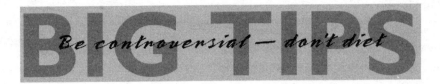

BIG TIPS *Be controversial — don't diet*

Imagine getting up, opening the wardrobe — and everything in there fits you. You look in the mirror, smile and decide what to wear from a selection of clothes that fit you and that you like. Wouldn't it feel great?

It's not normal to survive on only two or three outfits to wear. You're large and you're treating yourself as abnormal. But if you stay the same weight, then you can behave and shop like any 'normal' woman and, over a number of years, develop a mix-and-match wardrobe just like anyone else. Sounds good, doesn't it?

Diet Culture

Articles in the press repeatedly say that at any one time in this country, 60% of women are on a diet. Some attain their goal weight and stay slim for ever more — but the majority spend a lifetime yo-yoing up and down the scale.

Mary Evans Young is the founder of the UK-based organisation Diet Breakers, which she started to help women break free from the diet trap. She is also the originator of International No Diet Day, celebrated on 6 May each year. In her recent book, *Diet Breaking*, Mary produced some startling facts and figures:

- **96% of dieters regain all the weight they lose.** Most end up weighing more than when they started. *This means only four women out of every 100 maintain their weight loss.*
- **A high proportion of dieters control their weight by joining slimming clubs.** The bulk of slimming club membership is made up of comparatively slim women (sizes 14 to 18) trying to get slimmer. Although these clubs work for some, you can spend a fortune joining them. Women often attend weekly, stop for a while and then rejoin — and clubs use all sorts of wiles to encourage lapsed members back into the fold: cards, letters, phone calls and even little poems, to make the guilt nag at you until you succumb.
- **A survey of reduced-fat and low-fat foods in leading supermarkets, conducted in October 1994, found that manufacturers were charging up to 40% more for lower-fat equivalent products.**

Looking at these figures, I couldn't help thinking that the money women spend on diet foods and clubs would be much better spent on treating themselves to a new outfit to help them feel good the way they are.

Mending Your 'Appestat'

Most women whose weight has yo-yoed for years are terrified to stop dieting in case their weight just goes on escalating. My friend Yvonne is typical. She is 5ft 9in and veers between size 22 and size 16. When she's a 16, she really is quite slim for her height. Yvonne is now 52 and back to being a size 16. She has the proverbial wardrobe full of clothes and nothing to wear because everything is too big. She believes one of the main reasons for her weight fluctuations is that, like most large women, she has a 'fat' brain. She says she eats, breathes and thinks like a 'fat' person.

This set me thinking: what about all those non-dieting women who seem to eat whatever they want and stay a regulation size 12? How do their brains work?

Think about *your* non-dieting friends. I've been watching some of mine ever since Yvonne made that remark to me. They eat a lot when they are hungry and less when they are not. They recognise their appetite signals. Watch how these friends react to food. At a party they probably eat as much as you do, but the next day they subconsciously register that they ate a lot last night and automatically eat a little less — because their brain is tuned in to their bodily needs.

Many large women have lost this ability to regulate their eating. I call it a broken 'appestat' (like a thermostat for your appetite). Your 'appestat' should control your eating like a thermostat controls the heating in your house. We all have an 'appestat' in our brain, which regulates when and how to eat: we eat when we are hungry and stop when we're full. Only some people's appestat has stopped working in the normal pattern.

Think about going out for lunch. Today you are on a diet. You're not that hungry — what you really fancy is a pastry and a coffee or perhaps a lasagne. But you agreed with your 'fat' brain on Monday that *this* week you are going to diet. So you order a cottage cheese salad and a black coffee. Feeling extremely righteous you go back to work, and by mid-afternoon you are starving. But having been 'so good' at lunchtime you decline the proffered Mars bar. By the time you get home your stomach feels as if your throat has been cut and you binge on everything in sight while you cook dinner for the family. Does this sound familiar?

Alternatively, this is the week you are *not* dieting. You take yourself out for lunch. You are not particularly hungry and you're one of those rare women who actually likes cottage cheese. But you can't possibly order *that* — you're not on a diet this week. Instead you focus on the wonderful array of pastries and decide on the creamiest, jammiest one. Then, as you are *not* dieting, you order a lasagne to eat first and smother it with extra cheese.

You are behaving according to a diet mentality, not responding to what your body is telling you naturally. I want to show you how to think like a 'normal' person, eat and behave like a 'normal' person and develop a 'normal' appestat.

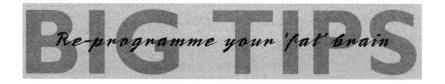

BIG TIPS

Re-programme your 'fat' brain

You are large and for you it is normal to be large. You know you like cottage cheese, you also like pastries. So be logical, eat like a 'normal' person would. On this occasion you're not particularly hungry, so either have cottage cheese for lunch or just a pastry. Or just have the lasagne. Choose whatever you actually feel like on the menu, without any regard to calorific value (the pastry and the lasagne are probably about equal calories and the cottage cheese a lot less, but pay no attention to that, eat what you want to eat).

Don't let choosing the pastry automatically put you into non-diet mode so that you have to have something else to prove to yourself that you are not dieting.

If you choose the cottage cheese because that's what you feel like eating, you will find it far more satisfying than if you choose it because it's a good diet food. The chances are that as you weren't hungry and you have eaten what you really fancied, you will not be starving by mid-afternoon. If you are, you can accept the Mars bar — and then you won't binge in the evening.

Jane Tyler is thirty-five years old and a size 20. She is a teacher, married to a solicitor, and has two teenage boys. Jane had a wardrobe stuffed full of clothes ranging from size 14 to size 22. However, she lived mainly in the same few outfits as they were the only ones that fitted. For the past ten years, once or twice each year, she has dieted and lost a stone, going down one size. Suddenly, she had another dozen outfits to wear for a few euphoric weeks. Then it would be back to her usual limited selection.

Some days she was happy with herself at a size 18. Other days she looked nostalgically at all the size 14 clothes she wore before she had the boys. This made her even more miserable. Then something would trigger off an eating binge and she would be back to a size 20 — and sometimes a size 22.

Two years ago she decided that enough was enough. I talked her through my appestat idea. It took her about six months to tune her 'fat' brain to the foods she really liked. Much to her surprise she discovered that although she loves sweet foods, she has a savoury palate too. During that six months her waistband fluctuated only marginally and she continued to live in her size 20s (though she wouldn't buy anything new). When the six months was up, we went on a shopping spree and she rid her wardrobe of all the clothes that were too small. She is still a size 20, but now so is everything in her wardrobe.

Fattist Society

The media has a lot to answer for when it comes to how women are viewed by society in general. Television, radio, magazines, advertising hoardings — everywhere we look we are bombarded with the message that it's not OK for a woman to be anything other than a size 10/12. The fashion industry has begun to make even women who are a size 12 feel that there is something wrong with them.

Have you ever noticed, for instance, how in 'before' and 'after' features, the 'before' picture is usually a family snap taken by an amateur, the woman looks a mess and it's taken at an unflattering angle; while in the 'after' photograph, she has suddenly met a professional photographer, her hair is freshly styled and she's wearing full make-up. I'd hazard a guess that the 'before' woman would have looked jolly nice anyway if she'd just been to the hairdresser and the beautician and had the benefit of a professional to take the shot.

Although there is an increasing awareness of the needs of larger women, we still live in a 'fattist' society.

For years I felt obliged always to be on a diet. Then one day, when someone asked me how much weight I had lost, I realised it was probably as much as thirty-two stone — the result of yo-yoing up and down the weight scale (lose three stone, gain four; lose five stone, gain three; lose four stone, gain five, and so on). And don't you just hate those weight/height charts? According to them, I'd probably be the right weight for my height if I were 8ft 3in.

In fact, it is possible to be large and perfectly in proportion. You may be big-boned, big-breasted or tall — being large does not automatically mean being fat. Recent research has shown that the average standard-size measurements for British women have increased significantly over the past forty years — waist and hip measurements by two inches on average; busts by one and a half inches; upper arms and ribcages are larger, too.

Despite this, children today are growing up surrounded by prejudices about diet and size. Children as young as six and seven are now dieting, in a world where, according to Mary Evans Young, 90% of women diet at some stage during their lifetime.

There are subtle messages everywhere. For example, the hit film *Home Alone* was sponsored by Diet Coke. This may seem a minor point— it's only a Cola, after all — but, very subtly, children are being encouraged to buy diet products like this at an ever earlier age. They are learning the diet mentality — to have a 'fat' attitude to food.

We are all born with a normal attitude to food. Babies suck when they are hungry and spit out the teat or nipple when they are full. They listen to their internal hunger cues. People who overeat need to relearn this ability to know when they are hungry and when they are not.

Why Do You Eat?

It is particularly important to differentiate between physical hunger and emotional hunger. You need to find a way other than eating to deal with your emotions.

Do you eat when you're unhappy or stressed? Do you use food as a comforter? Is eating the way you avoid dealing with problems? Those problems will still be there when you finish that last mouthful.

From now on, each time you eat, think about why you are eating and whether you have any alternatives...

- **Bored?** ... Do something — read a book, write a letter, go for a walk, make a phone call. If you don't feel like doing any of these and the urge to eat is too strong, at least go for a walk round the block first. Who knows, you might bump into a friend and get side-tracked.

- **Tired?** ... Have a rest — sit down and relax with a coffee for five minutes; if there's time, take a bath. If you're too busy now to take a break, promise yourself one at a set time.

- **Angry?** ... Shout! If you can't shout at the person you want to and you have a car, take a drive — close all the windows, pretend that person is on the back seat and shout and scream at them to your heart's content. Alternatively, try shouting and screaming in the shed at the bottom of the garden, or — when the house is empty — in the bathroom.

- **Lonely?** ... Phone somebody, write a letter, go for a walk, listen to the radio (perhaps join in one of the chat shows), watch TV.

- **Stressed?** ...Slow down, relax, treat yourself — a massage, manicure, hairdo (if you haven't time, diary some time for yourself and make do with a bunch of flowers, a magazine or CD for now); have a relaxing bath.

- **Socialising?** ... If you're hungry, eat. If you're not hungry but want to be sociable, join in, but don't overdo it.

- **Frustrated?** ... Try to define why, and work out how to do something about it.
- **In a hurry?** ... You'll have more time to get the work done if you forget the food.
- **Need comforting?** ... Ask someone for a cuddle — even if it's only the dog; confide in a close friend.
- **Sad?** ... Try to deal with why you are feeling sad and find something to do to lift the mood.
- **Happy?** ... Focus on the happiness itself and really get enjoyment from that feeling — then you shouldn't crave food.
- **Can't sleep?** ... Have a bath, perhaps using a relaxing aromatherapy oil, listen to the radio, make a warm drink, do the crossword.
- **Hungry?** ... Fine — eat and enjoy. STOP when you are full, and only eat the food you really feel like. However, think again whether you are actually physically hungry or if any of the emotional excuses above apply. Only eat when you are really physically hungry (find out how you can tell the difference in the quiz below).

Are You Really Hungry?

What if you've got out of the habit of recognising real hunger cues? Try thinking of hunger on a scale of one to ten, as set out below. Preferably only eat when you are at levels three and four. When your hunger level is under five you are eating because you are physically hungry. Once you eat when your level is five or above you are eating because of an emotion. It's also important to try not to let your hunger level sink as low as levels one and two.

ONE TO TEN / HUNGER LEVEL SCALE

(adapted from *You Count, Calories Don't* by Mary Evans Young)

ONE   If you have ever fasted, it's how you feel after about twenty hours without food:

- You probably have a headache — if not, you feel quite light-headed
- You feel dizzy and can't think straight
- You have no energy and would prefer to be lying down
- You may have trouble with your co-ordination

TWO   If you usually eat breakfast and lunch, it's how you feel at 2p.m. when all you've had is a coffee:

- You're in a filthy mood
- You have no patience for anyone or anything
- You're so hungry you feel you could eat anything in sight
- You feel you have no energy
- Your stomach keeps rumbling
- You're not sure if you want to eat or be sick

THREE This is how you feel when you haven't had a chance to have a snack or a nibble and it's four hours since your last decent meal:

- Your concentration is not all it should be
- Your stomach feels empty
- The urge to eat is strong

FOUR   How you feel after a couple of hours without food — when, if you were offered a snack or a three course meal, you might take the snack:

- You're aware that you are a little hungry
- You're aware it's some while since you ate anything
- You begin to wonder what to nibble at

FIVE– Another couple of mouthfuls and you will feel full up

FIVE   This is the point at which people with a 'normal' attitude to food stop eating:

- You are not hungry any more
- You are physically and psychologically satisfied

FIVE+   This is when people with a diet mentality continue to eat:

- You are eating more than you need
- You are feeding your emotional hunger — really think about why you are eating now

SIX   You're past being full up — yet you could still eat some more (your mother probably would have said 'your eyes are bigger than your belly'):

- Your body says 'no' … your mind says 'just a little bit more'

SEVEN   You probably need to loosen your belt:

- You feel uncomfortable
- You need a break before you eat some more

EIGHT   You're beyond feeling full:

- You are eating for the sake of something to do
- You are actually starting to hurt

NINE   You've dieted all week to have this 'blow-out' and now you feel positively ill:

- You feel heavy
- You feel tired
- You need to go home and lie down

TEN   You're either on your annual holiday or it's Christmas and you're on a two-week binge:

- You'll be pleased when the holiday's over so that you can eat less
- You go to bed feeling ill
- You get up feeling bloated
- You keep promising yourself that you won't eat for a week once this holiday is over

If you recognised your own over-eating pattern here and want to regain control of your eating, weight and life without dieting, Mary Evans Young's book *You Count, Calories Don't* is well worth reading.

When choosing what to eat, remember not to think in terms of diet or non-diet labels. Then you can decide on the basis of whether you like the flavours. If you like salads, don't think of them as rabbit food but as something you enjoy.

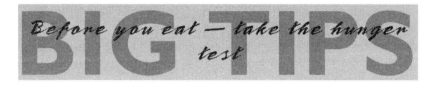

Before you eat — take the hunger test

However, allowing yourself to eat without 'diet' restrictions doesn't mean you can go mad. Don't smother a salad with dollops of mayonnaise that you know full well are highly calorific — after all, you want to stay the same size, not expand. That said, you can still dress your salad in moderation with a real dressing that you find delicious — not a diet dressing, which is often either so synthetically sweet or so sour that it takes away the enjoyment of the entire meal.

If you love chips, that's fine too. Obviously if you have a huge portion with every meal you won't achieve your objective of staying the same size. But once or twice a week allow yourself an average portion and don't feel guilty — *enjoy them*.

Do you find the idea of eating this way frightening? The only way to see if it works is to try it. If diets don't work for

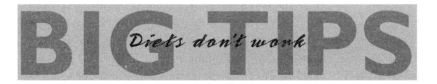

Diets don't work

you, give this approach a try for at least six months, preferably a year (it really does take that long to get out of the diet mentality). You'll soon be able to tell if it isn't working because your waistbands will get tighter. But I really doubt that this will happen.

Throw Out the Scales

If you are one of those women who weighs yourself daily — DON'T. It is soul-destroying.

Brenda, a client who has been an anorexic size 6, a bulimic size 24 and is now a contented size 18, used to do just that. She has four children and works part time, book-keeping for her husband, an electrician. She would weigh herself as soon as she woke up; after

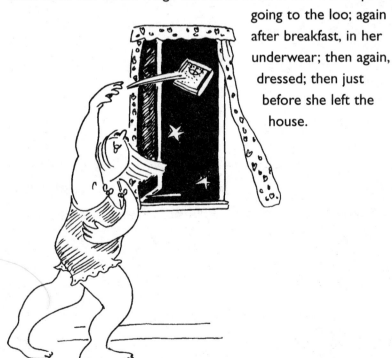

going to the loo; again after breakfast, in her underwear; then again, dressed; then just before she left the house.

When she came home, the first thing she did was step on the scales … then go to the loo and weigh herself again… She was aware how obsessive this was but found it impossible to stop. If her weight was down, it was a 'good' day and she could resist her favourite foods. If her weight was up, she would try to resist, but would usually end up having a 'bad' day, and binge. The next day would be a struggle to decide whether it would be a 'good' or a 'bad' day. Although Brenda knew that the fluctuations in her weight often related to her moods rather than the food she had eaten, her weight fluctuations still affected how good or bad she felt about herself.

When I first met Brenda, she was a size 20. We talked about her giving herself 'permission' to stay large and we went shopping for some clothes in her size. She then gave me her scales to lock in the boot of my car. For the first couple of weeks she found it very hard to live without them, then suddenly it became an immense relief. The waistband of her clothes was a much better indication of weight fluctuation. And, as predicted, Brenda is now taking one size smaller. The size 20 clothes that she bought have been taken in or, where the style still looks good, she is wearing them that bit looser.

The waistband test is much better than constantly weighing yourself. It's an accurate enough reflection of any size increase, without making you obsessively aware of fractional changes. Bear in mind, though, that around your period your waistbands may feel a little tighter, but the following week they will be fine again.

Now or Never

You may know that you don't stand a chance of ever being slim enough to wear some of the clothes in your wardrobe again, but you still can't bear to get rid of them. Or perhaps you have a collection of clothes which very *nearly* fit you. Or even some that you do wear that are a bit tight, but if you breathe in ... And last of all perhaps you have one or two items that actually fit you and that you don't feel too bad in.

Maybe it's time to accept yourself as you are. In fact, *it's now or never time ...*

I want you to really look at yourself properly. Perhaps it will be for the first time for many years. The main reason women diet is low self-esteem. Your awareness of being large overshadows all your good points. 'What good points?' some of you will say. Try this exercise.

The 'Long, Hard Look' Test

At the earliest opportunity, preferably when everyone else is out, do your hair, put on a little make-up and stand in front of a mirror — and it must be a full-length one — in bra and pants. Then evaluate every part of your body ticking the 'good', 'average' and 'not so good' boxes in the chart overleaf.

Now look through the list. Every woman has more good points than she realises. Even if you only tick one 'good' you have a feature you can make the most of.

You haven't ticked any good points? I'm sorry, I don't believe you. Do the test again — there must be at least one good point you can tick. And if there still isn't, smile at yourself until you have to tick that one.

Decide now to be satisfied with the parts of you that you have ticked as good and as average. This is what you like about yourself. Later in the book I will help you understand how to dress to highlight your good points and minimise the areas you are not happy about.

HIGHLIGHT YOUR GOOD POINTS

	Good	Average	Not so good
Hair	☐	☐	☐
Make-up	☐	☐	☐
Skin	☐	☐	☐
Eyes	☐	☐	☐
Nose	☐	☐	☐
Ears	☐	☐	☐
Mouth	☐	☐	☐
Smile	☐	☐	☐
Posture	☐	☐	☐
Neck	☐	☐	☐
Shoulders	☐	☐	☐
Arms	☐	☐	☐
Hands	☐	☐	☐
Nails	☐	☐	☐
Cleavage	☐	☐	☐
Bust	☐	☐	☐
Waist	☐	☐	☐
Hips	☐	☐	☐
Thighs	☐	☐	☐
Knees	☐	☐	☐
Legs	☐	☐	☐
Ankles	☐	☐	☐
Feet	☐	☐	☐
Toes	☐	☐	☐

But first, physical attributes aside, what do you think of your overall image? Or do you not think of it at all? A positive self-image works wonders for your self-esteem. Try this short exercise to see how you rate various aspects of your image.

How Well Do You Come Across?

Assess your image

Look at the different elements of how you come across to other people below and give yourself marks on a scale of 1 to 5 for each one:

- **Making conversation**
- **Eye contact and body language**
- **Making friends**
- **Personality**
- **Grooming (hair, skin, etc.)**
- **Manners**
- **Fitness**

Score 1 Terrible. Needs lots of attention.

Score 2 Not your greatest asset. Could use some work.

Score 3 OK some of the time, but improvement wouldn't hurt.

Score 4 Usually pretty good, but perhaps not perfect.

Score 5 Excellent; this is always spot on.

Scoring

Less than 10? Oh dear! You either have a lot of hard work ahead of you to improve your overall image, or you're very underconfident of your own abilities.

10–18? You need to polish up in some areas, but it's perfectly possible with just a little effort.

Did you score between 19 and 27? Your overall image is good. Keep working at any weak spots, though.

Did you score over 28? Are you perfect? Or did you cheat?

I cover ways to improve all these aspects of your image in later chapters, so remember which areas needed special attention as you read on.

Men Like Big Women Who Like Themselves

Every woman, of any size, deserves to have an excellent self-image. How you feel about yourself and your body has an impact on every area of your life: your confidence at work, your friendships, and, particularly, your relationships. Many large women who are single blame the fact that they can't find a man on their size. If you think that you are never going to find a partner because you're big — think again.

Josie used to be a permanently hungry, unhappy size 10; she is now a contented size 20/22. 'My husband likes me big,' she says, 'he doesn't like skinny women. He didn't tell me at the time, but now he says that when I was slim it was like making love to a lamppost — my hipbones used to grind against him! I'm so happy with myself now that I no longer diet. I am what I am. I carry myself well, I like to make a dramatic entrance, I walk tall and feel proud of myself.'

Corinne is 5ft 5in and a size 26; she has been married three times and I have never seen her without a man in tow. She says, 'Lots of men have a fantasy of being surrounded and lost in a mountain of flesh — not many women can make their wish come true.'

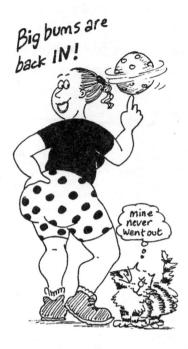

Marilyn is 5ft 3in and size 18, she is now 43 and has never married. Finding a partner has never been on her agenda, but she is rarely without a man at her side. She seems to attract men like bees round a honey-pot. She has a bubbly sense of humour and always looks amazing.

Isabel is 5ft 4in and a size 26; she told me 'I used to feel fat and ugly when I was single and then, when I realised my weight was a medical problem, I gradually came to terms with it. My family love me the way I am, my friends love me and say I wouldn't be me if I was skinny. I always make the most of the way I look, I have my hair cut regularly, I always wear make-up. It's important to me to like the way that I look before I leave the house.'

The majority of women who are contented with their man take a great deal of care with their appearance — they look good, exude confidence and are amazed at the audacity of anyone suggesting that their weight could affect their relationships.

You shouldn't have to dress to impress other people, you should be dressing to like what you see in the mirror. When a woman looks well put-together, most men will first see a woman who cares about herself. The fact that she is large becomes a secondary factor.

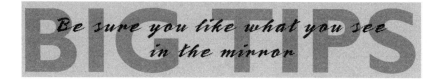

Be sure you like what you see
in the mirror

Remember that there are plenty of women out there who are not large and have difficulty finding the right man too. So you obviously can't blame your lack of men friends entirely on your size.

I called this section 'men like big women who like themselves', but it would be just as appropriate to say 'men like women who like themselves'. Food for thought?

Fit for Life

Now you know something about your own image, why and how you eat and how important it is to feel happy about your size. Next I'm going to discuss another sometimes touchy subject for large women — health and fitness. Many large women think they aren't fit, because they're told they can't be, at their size. And, obviously, you're never going to be happy with your weight, or buy clothes in the right size to fit you now, if you feel you *have* to diet constantly for your health. So in the next chapter, I aim to show that it is possible to be large *and* healthy.

CHAPTER TWO

Big and Healthy

'IT IS POSSIBLE TO BE FAT AND FIT'

Over and over again, when I discuss staying large with large women, they tell me, 'I need to lose weight because it's unhealthy to be this size.' While it's true that for some medical conditions, such as diabetes or high blood pressure, losing weight can often help, there's a whole host of illnesses for which being large is unfairly blamed. As many slim people as large ones have painful joints, osteoporosis, heart problems, bad backs and so on. In many cases, it's healthier for a person to be large than to diet constantly. In any event, losing weight permanently is a long, slow process, which doesn't usually come about through dieting. It is more likely to happen naturally, and long-term, if you can develop a healthy relationship with food and your body.

Diet Damage

Here's some food for thought. An article in the *Daily Mail* in June 1996 claimed that dieting can reduce your brain power. Some people who were actually slimming when they performed tests of memory, reaction speeds and ability to sustain high concentration levels achieved worse results than those who were happy with their weight (whatever it was). According to Dr. Mike Green, who did this research originally for *Which? Health* magazine, dieters are so obsessed with following a strict regime that they endure high levels of stress and anxiety, which soak up much of their mental energy.

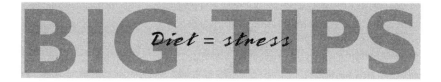

This may sound far-fetched, but think about it. Dieters spend nearly every waking moment thinking about food — deciding what you can eat which is low in calories but will fill you up; or wondering what you can binge on, because you're not dieting that week. Stress levels mount with each passing day.

Escaping the Trap

There *is* a way out, however. Instead of tormenting yourself with dreams of forbidden foods, just *stop* thinking about diets or calories altogether. Focus on food you genuinely like that you know is also nutritious — *ordinary* food that you can cook for yourself and the family. How would that feel? Liberating? I assure you, you will be far less stressed and find you have much more mental energy to cope with everyday living.

Take Jean and Marion, for example. I've known Jean for three years and Marion is one of Jean's school friends whom I recently met. Marion was on a diet, which led me to chat to them both about their bodies and their weight.

Jean is 5ft 8in, 49 years old and a size 20. Her battle with her weight started at school. She was the tallest in her class and always felt large and clumsy. Now, Jean realises that she was probably not even fat, just a sturdy size 14; but she was conscious of being taller and bigger all over than everyone else in her class. Unfortunately for her, at that time, the skinny model, Twiggy, and fashions that suited her stick-like body were all the rage, making Jean feel unfashionable and *fat*.

Marion was astounded by Jean's comments; she recalled her having a nice figure at school. Jean's mother didn't help: she made Jean more self-conscious about her size by putting her on the Mayo Diet, which was protein, salad, fruit and not a lot else. 'I am sure that if I hadn't dieted so severely all those years ago, I wouldn't be the size that I am today,' she says now. 'I hated every minute of it and must have dieted my metabolism into a dreadful state.'

Jean was a temporary size 12 when she met and married Robert. He fell for her as a blonde nymphet and liked her to dress in provocative styles. She never really felt comfortable with this and, after three children in quick succession, she no longer fitted the picture at all. Robert demoralised her by going out with other women, implying that it was her fault. 'You're so fat, how could I fancy you now?' he'd say.

When she tried to talk to him about separation he would taunt her, 'How are you ever going to get a life without me?' and 'No one will ever want you — you're too fat'.

By the time they finally divorced, Jean had a totally negative self-image and forced herself to join a dieting club. Her weight fluctuated for years. She would lose weight, buy new clothes, stay slim for a while, then pile it all on again — each time at least a half a stone more than before. About ten years ago, when Jean reached the weight she is today, she simply decided that she didn't want to put on any more weight — and the only way to do that was *never* to diet again. She also decided it was time for another man in her life, but this time she didn't want to diet in order to date. 'I wanted to find a man who would like me the way I would always be. Not to diet and then have to stay that way to please a man. I like me as I am — I wanted to find a man who would like me this way too.'

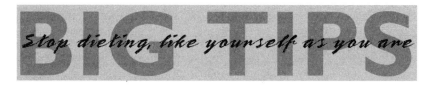

BIG TIPS

Stop dieting, like yourself as you are

She knew she'd found her man when she was on holiday in America with Robert (mark II). They dropped into a coffee house for a snack and Jean said she fancied pancakes, described on the menu as being smothered in maple syrup and cream.

'Pancakes for two,' Robert said to the skinny waitress.

'She doesn't need 'em,' said the waitress. 'She'd better share yours or have a salad.'

'Thank you very much,' retaliated Robert, 'but the lady and I will both have pancakes — and don't be mean with the cream.'

Marion couldn't be more of a contrast to Jean. She is a five foot, bubbly, bouncy blonde. At school, she was a cute, elfin size 8 — a real Sixties' babe. She wore mini skirts and hot pants — 'the tighter and shorter, the better'. Today she is a size 18 and perpetually on a diet. She fluctuates from size 14 to size 20. Even when she's a size 14, she still strives for her ultimate dream of being size 8 again, although in everyone else's eyes she looks gorgeous. She's happily married, and her husband, children and grandchildren adore her. Despite that, Marion's whole life is dominated by what she ate yesterday, what she ate this morning and what she'll eat for the rest of the day.

Wouldn't you agree that it is mentally so much healthier to be like Jean, happy with her size and weight, than like Marion, who is constantly striving to be something that is no longer natural for her body?

Look After Your Heart

You will hear it stressed time and again that being overweight is bad for your health. Of course, it's best to find your natural, healthy body weight by eating a well-balanced diet and adopting an active lifestyle. But that's not the same thing as *having* to be slim. You should be developing your confidence and self-esteem; making the most of yourself and getting on with life, not dieting to achieve some elusive 'perfect' weight. However, women who find the idea of not dieting hard to accept can perhaps take comfort from the fact that there is some evidence that dieting can actually damage your heart more than staying large. Shelley Bovey, in her book *The Forbidden Body — Why Being Fat is Not a Sin*, writes this:

> Several large companies in the United States have stopped urging their employees to lose weight and, instead, introduced programmes advocating self-acceptance, healthy eating and a complete disregard for weighing scales.

There were several factors involved in that about-turn. Some important long-term studies were published which looked at the effects and the effectiveness of dieting. They all demonstrated that diets do not work. What's more, persistent yo-yo dieting was cited as a far greater risk of premature death than being overweight. Among groups monitored over a period of many years, even those who grew significantly fat lived longer than those who repeatedly dieted and then regained; a margin of as little as 11lbs either way was cited as being risky.

...weight lost is nearly always regained; weight recycling (yo-yo dieting) is harmful; the various weight loss methods on offer were ineffectual and actually caused harm. Most important of all, the government acknowledged that most major studies suggested that increased mortality is associated with weight loss.

...Another aspect of the recent research has thrown up the startling information that many heart attacks occurring in large people and previously attributed to their obesity were found to have occurred while those individuals were in the process of losing weight. On autopsy some were found to have died due to loss of heart muscle.

We are constantly told that being overweight increases your blood pressure. However, studies suggest it's more likely that it is not the actual being overweight that causes higher blood pressure, but the stress of continually dieting and yo-yoing in weight which is the culprit.

According to Janice Bhend, Editor of YES! magazine, 'There is no concrete evidence that being large is bad for your heart. The so-called experts are always preaching doom and gloom, but if you have a healthy lifestyle and your heart is used to carrying that extra weight, your heart learns to cope with it and accommodates you at the weight you are. When you lose weight too quickly the heart can't cope and this can result in a heart attack. Also, when you lose weight you lose bone mass as well (particularly after the menopause), and this can result in osteoporosis. Load bearing (such as excess weight) on bones keeps them strong.'

Backs and Bones

I spoke to a chiropractor, Dr. Sandra Richer, about the implications of being large on back pain and other related skeletal problems. I asked her if large people have more back problems. In Dr. Richer's opinion, a bad back is rarely directly caused by a weight problem. Statistically, two out of five people will have back pain in their life time. People who regularly do heavy physical work are less inclined to injure their backs because their backs are stronger, but when they do suffer an injury it is usually more severe. Sedentary people have more of a tendency to back pain than people who are physically fit because they are not exercising their muscles enough.

Dr. Richer told me that losing weight in itself does not cure a bad back and, in any event, *there are as many slim people as large people with bad backs.* 'Unfortunately,' she added, 'we live in a world built for the average person. If you are taller than average, you tend to stoop frequently and this can cause back problems. If you are shorter, you frequently overstretch and this can be just as bad. But when a big person consults a doctor about back pain, too often the doctor makes the assumption that it is the weight that is causing the pain. The most common answer the average doctor gives to a patient about back pain is, "lose weight, exercise, diet".

'In my opinion, however,' Dr. Richer said, 'if you are in acute pain, until you are actually out of pain you aren't going to be able to exercise, and if you are in constant pain, how are you going to have the initiative to diet and lose weight?'

BIG TIPS
Diets don't cure back pain

Dr. Richer explained that she first treats the problem, say acute back pain or perhaps arthritis, and *then* looks at diet and other factors. 'Joint problems, when people are carrying a lot of extra weight proportionately, depend on height and how the weight is carried. The most common weight-related problem is wear and tear of joints such as the knee joint.'

A lot of large women are also very busty and this can cause mid-back pain — a good bra can make the world of difference.

I asked her opinion on corsets. Her answer was that many women of sixty-five plus have been wearing corsets for years, and as a result their back muscles have become weak and they now need the corset permanently. Her view is that a corset can give invaluable support if back pain is acute but it is not a good idea in the long term, because of this reliance that develops.

Bad posture also has a lot to do with back problems, as does how long you have been large and how quickly you put the weight on. Says Dr. Richer, 'A big weight gain over a short time puts more of a strain on the spine.'

The best exercise for your back is swimming, recommended by the majority of chiropractors and osteopaths, though some doctors advise you not to swim on your front if back pain is severe. There are many different opinions on this, but Dr. Richer's advice is to avoid breast stroke when back pain is acute, then, as your back mends, to introduce it as *one* of your strokes. 'Breast stroke,' she added, 'is a form of extension exercise and this type of stretching isn't a good idea for a patient in acute pain — it can exacerbate the problem. But once past the acute stage, extension exercises are a good idea as they increase mobility.'

Many people also find the Alexander technique very helpful for improving posture and easing backache. An increasing number of health clubs and leisure centres offer classes in the technique, and it is a good alternative for those who cannot, or would rather not, swim.

Although Dr. Richer agrees that one positive thing about carrying those extra pounds is that you are less likely to suffer from osteoporosis, she emphasises that this is rather a sweeping generalisation. 'If you have a family history of osteoporosis, if you have been anorexic or starved at any point, if you don't have periods or you have a very early menopause, these things will work against you, but generally large women are less prone to osteoporosis because they continually exert more pressure on their weight-bearing joints. And light weight-bearing exercises strengthen the bones.'

The Pleasure Principle

If you're not entirely convinced, there's a lot more evidence that weight and ill-health don't necessarily go hand in hand.

According to a recent article in the *Daily Mail,* an international survey by the Association of Research into the Science of Enjoyment (ARISE) looked at attitudes in eight different countries towards thirteen everyday pleasures. These included eating cakes and ice cream, chocolate, cheese, cream and butter; drinking beer, wine and spirits, tea and coffee; and eating out. Here are some of its conclusions:

> ARISE founder Professor David Warburton, head of psychopharmacology at the University of Reading, said, 'People really should not feel guilty about pleasure-giving activities, as long as they don't over-indulge or harm others. Guilt acts as an important social check on personal behaviour... in its extreme, guilt can impair attentiveness, making people forgetful and more prone to error. Chronic guilt can induce stress and depression which could lead to eating disorders and contribute to infection, ulcers, heart problems and even brain damage.' His colleague Dr. Neil Sherwood added, 'A favourite treat reduces stress and helps people relax.'

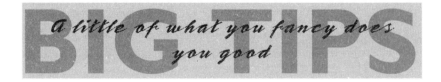

A little of what you fancy does you good

And Dr. Jill Wellborne of the Eating Disorders Clinic at the Bristol Royal Infirmary is quoted in *YES!* magazine as follows:

> Overweight per se is not a health risk. Nor are there any associated problems with pregnancy and overweight. Serious overweight — where you really cannot do your

shoes up — is different, but even then weight should not be lost by dieting. Permanent, pleasant lifestyle changes should be made (in other words — we should all be eating a diet high in complex carbohydrates, fruit and vegetables and low in fat, and we should be taking more exercise)… Lack of cardio-respiratory (heart-lung) fitness is due to lack of exercise and should not be attributed to obesity. If you eat well and take exercise — regular brisk walking is good — then you can *enjoy good health at any weight.*.' (my italics).

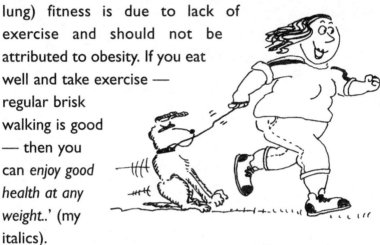

Jill stresses that whatever your weight, you are safer staying there than losing and regaining. 'It's no good going from 20 stone to 16 — and back up again,' she says. 'Unless you can be sure of losing weight very slowly, and keeping it off permanently without dieting, don't do it. You'd be daft to try.'

A Giant Leap

I hope that the information in this chapter has convinced you never to diet again. I want you to be at ease with the idea of eating normally, taking exercise and feeling healthy. Now you're in the right frame of mind to learn how to make the most of the person you are. Read on!

CHAPTER THREE

Taking the Plunge

'WOMEN WEAR 15% OF THEIR CLOTHES 85% OF THE TIME'

*I*n the average woman's wardrobe there is a vast collection of clothes in a dazzling variety of colours and styles. Many of them won't have been worn for at least a year and some have never been worn at all. Research shows that we wear 15% of our clothes 85% of the time.

Look in any large woman's wardrobe and you find not only the normal mish-mash of shapes and shades, but also a wide range of sizes, which restricts the choice of what can actually be worn at any one time even further.

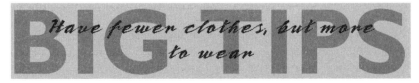

BIG TIPS

Have fewer clothes, but more to wear

If you recognise the description and are laughing wryly, then this chapter is written with you in mind. It will show you how to organise your wardrobe and develop a versatile and well co-ordinated collection of clothes. This chapter explains the process. If you're not sure how to find the right clothes for your body shape and individual colouring, the following chapters will help. With my system, you'll probably end up buying fewer clothes — so you'll have more money to spend on the right ones. Instead of owning a wardrobe full of clothes but nothing to wear, you'll soon have a wardrobe which is only half full... *but wear everything in it.*

First Impressions

First of all, just a little persuasion to convince you that you *do* want to overhaul your wardrobe. 'You can't judge a book by its cover' has a lot of truth in it — but if you hadn't liked the cover of this book, would you even have looked at it, let alone bought it, in the first place? Likewise, you know the expression 'You only get one chance to make a first impression' is obviously true, too. We all tend to sum up the people we meet within a few seconds, before they have uttered a word; we make assumptions about their financial position, social status, integrity, professionalism and even level of education just from what they look like.

Your appearance and how you act are non-verbal forms of communication. According to US psychologist Albert Mehrabian, statistically others will sum you up as follows:

55% is the way you look
38% is the way you act
7% is what you actually have to say

To ensure that you are your own best asset at all times you need to know how to make the most of that vital 55% *and* 38% — a vast 93% of a first impression.

That 93% relates to the way you look, your body language, how you move and the way you obviously feel about yourself. It's imperative that the first impression is not just good, but excellent.

When you know you look good, you feel good and it shows. And when that first impression is impressive, people will want to listen to you and will pay heed to what you say — that final 7%. I can't teach you what to say, although this is probably the most important aspect to *you* — when you speak, you're on your own. But I hope I can help you a lot with the 93% — your visual presentation. The clothes you wear play an important role in this.

Wardrobe for a Lifestyle

Before you can effectively reorganise your wardrobe you need to evaluate your lifestyle and look at your existing clothes collection critically. I'm going to help you with five projects I have devised. You'll need to devote some time to them, and you may find some parts a little hard to do, but your reward will be knowing that you are doing something constructive about improving your image.

Project one — analyse your lifestyle

Look through your diary for the last year and see what activities take up most of your time. Assuming that you spend six to eight hours a day in bed (did I hear you say, 'I wish'?), and the remaining sixteen to eighteen hours dressed, look at how many hours a day/week/year you spend on the following activities:

- **Commuting**
- **Working**
- **Doing the school run**
- **Shopping**
- **Housework**
- **Hobbies**
- **Socialising**

From this, divide your lifestyle into appropriate style categories such as :

- CASUAL/SPORTY Walking the dog, going to the gym, school run
- CASUAL/SMART Work (for some people), lunch with friends, shopping locally
- SMART (DAYTIME) Work (for some people), business meetings, meeting teachers, shopping in town
- SMART (EVENING) Restaurant, theatre, cocktail party, dinner with friends
- GLAMOUR Black tie functions, dinner dances

— or invent your own categories to suit your lifestyle.

Really analyse your lifestyle carefully, and then evaluate your existing wardrobe. Does it reflect where you spend most of your time? Do you have suitable clothes for each category? Don't forget, your lifestyle will change and you will need to re-evaluate if you:

- **Stop work to have a baby**
- **Go back to working part time after having a baby**
- **Climb the career ladder** ...

Project two — match your wardrobe to your lifestyle
With the help of the lists you made in project one, I want you to draw yourself a 'pie-chart'. Mark off a slice of pie for each of your categories of activity — the bigger the slice, the more time you spend on that activity. Don't worry about being strictly accurate, but the relative size of your slices should be a good, visual indication of which activities take up the biggest slices of your life.

Here's mine ...

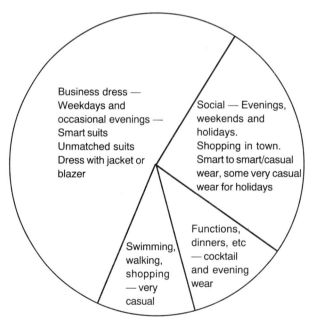

I spend a considerable number of hours each day with clients, and that is reflected in my pie chart. If I am with corporate clients in their offices, I wear a smart suit. With private clients in my studio at home, I am smart; I wear a jacket but not necessarily a suit. Socially, I prefer a more casual but quite smart look. I swim a couple of times a week and walk the dog daily so I need some really casual clothes too. I also have a few glamour functions to attend, so that takes up a chunk of my chart as well.

Now fill in yours ...

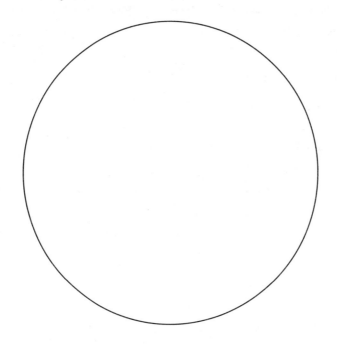

Now look at your pie chart and *really* take in where you are spending your hours and make sure that from now on, *you spend most money in the category where you spend most time.*

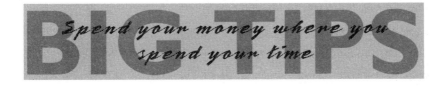

Spend your money where you spend your time

Interlude

While you gather your strength for the next project, here is a story to encourage you. Are you like my friend Gillian in this story?

For any occasion other than work Gillian gets dressed, looks in her mirror, gets undressed, discards the clothes on the bed and puts something else on. Another look in the mirror and she gets changed again. Of course, everthing she tries looks just as awful to her, so she ends up digging out in disgust the very first outfit she rejected and throwing it on — leaving in an extremely bad mood because she's late and doesn't have time to clear up the mountain of mess on her bed.

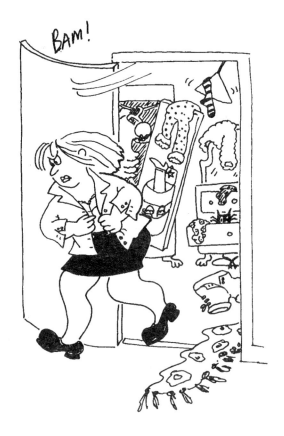

A client of mine, Rosemary, used to be like Gillian, but since accomplishing all the projects I'm giving you, the scenario is different. When Rosemary is going out, it doesn't take her long to decide what to wear. She likes, and knows she looks good in, everything in her wardrobe. When she's getting dressed, if the blouse or sweater she had in mind needs ironing or is in the wash, it really doesn't matter because all her clothes mix and match, so there's always something else that will be suitable. Does that spur you on? Move on to the next project!

Project three — weed your wardrobe

Put aside a couple of hours, half a day or a whole day, depending on how many clothes you have. Now, this time you have to be very strict with yourself — you're not particularly going to enjoy this. But, once you have done it thoroughly you will never have to do it so painfully again, because I am also going to show you a way to deal with your wardrobe in the future which will take you less than an hour, just twice a year.

This is the sort of job you have to get stuck into. You will welcome disturbances *so make sure you don't get any.* If you live on your own, put on the answerphone or take the phone off the hook and don't answer the front door. If you live with a friend, partner or anyone else, insist that they don't disturb you.

You should complete this project *before* you read the chapters on colour and style. I don't want you to be influenced by anything except your present attitude to the clothes in your wardrobe. There could be items you like in spite of the fact that you may find out later that they are not the best style or colour for you. That's fine, you keep them.

BIG TIPS
Rules are for bending

Later you can read the rules and see how you can bend them to make any colour and most styles work successfully for you. This project is not intended to strip your wardrobe of anything you really like. So, here's how to go about weeding your wardrobe.

Take each item out of your wardrobe and look hard at it. Ask yourself:

- **Do you like yourself in it?**
- **Do you think it suits you?**
- **Does it fit you?**
- **When did you last wear it?**

According to your answers, begin to put your clothes into four piles, as follows.

PILE ONE Clothes you *do* like yourself in, that you do wear, that you do think suit you. Put these, with pride, in a pile on the bed. This is the most important pile.

PILE TWO Clothes you know are old-fashioned or have passed their 'sell by' date. Turn them into cash by taking them to a car boot sale or give them to a charity shop (neatly folded, please!).

PILE THREE Clothes you haven't worn for a year or more because you:

- **Know they're out-of-date**, but think they may come back into fashion.

- **Still can't get into them**, however much you breathe in.
- **Know they are too big for you** (unless you like them and they are worth altering, then they go into pile four).
- **Never really liked them** from the moment you took them out of the bag.
- **Know they are the wrong colour or shape for you.**
- **Just never wear them and don't really know why.**
- **Know they don't go with anything else in your wardrobe**

Take this pile to a car boot sale or a charity shop, or give them to friends. If they are modern, hardly worn and in good condition, recycle them through a dress agency. Spend any proceeds on some really good clothes that will form part of your new wardrobe.

DIRE WARNING: Don't, under any circumstances, put anything from piles two and three back in your wardrobe. If you are a hoarder, find somewhere else to put them: a spare wardrobe, an empty suitcase, in the loft or in boxes under the bed. Anywhere, in fact, just so long as it is not your wardrobe.

If you find yourself reluctant to part with any of pile three, look again at your reasons for hoarding them.

- **They may come back into fashion.** True, they just might — but they rarely look as good second time around.

56 BIG LIVING

- **You can't get into them, however much you breathe in, but you just might, one day** ... GET THEM OUT OF YOUR WARDROBE. It's absolutely soul-destroying to have them hanging there. I don't care which pile they go into or what you do with them, so long as they are not dangling where you see them daily, to make you feel bad about yourself and your size.
- **They are too big for you, but you might, unfortunately, need them again.** OK, I do understand, but please keep them somewhere else, not in your wardrobe.
- **You never really liked them, but they are still practically as new.** It's very unlikely that you ever will like them, so why are you keeping them?
- **If you know they're the wrong colour or shape for you, you just never wear them and don't really know why, or they don't go with anything else in your wardrobe** — what's your problem? Why give them house room? By the end of this book, you'll understand your shape and colouring and why certain clothes don't suit you and others do.

PILE FOUR Anything you're not wearing because it:

- **needs shortening**
- **needs lengthening**
- **needs taking in**
- **has loose buttons**
- **has a hem coming undone**

From now on think of items like these as your pending wardrobe. If you haven't made the necessary repairs to these clothes within ten days, *they join piles two and three.*

Once you've dealt with pile four, decide on a permanent place for your pending wardrobe from now on, such as hanging on the outside of your wardrobe, on the ironing board or in a corner in the kitchen. *Never* put it back in your current wardrobe. I keep my pending wardrobe by the side of the chair where I watch TV as this reminds me to do the odd sewing jobs while watching my favourite programmes. The sewing that I can't do myself, and the dry cleaning, gets slung over the upstairs banister until I have time to take it to the cleaners or to my local alteration lady. I find this an effective ploy as it's an annoying sight and makes me remember to take it out with me.

Weed Accessories Too

It's important that your accessories, underwear and make-up get the same tough treatment. Here's how you do it:

SHOES First sort out the old-fashioned ones (these can really date you). If you want to keep them in case the fashion comes around again, banish them to the loft. Are there any shoes that you haven't worn for years because they're uncomfortable? Why are you keeping them? They're not suddenly going to become comfortable are they?

HANDBAGS Just keep the ones that you like, use regularly and that go with all your clothes. Are you ever going to use that lime green one that matched a pair of shoes you discarded years ago? I suspect the answer is no — so get rid of it.

SCARVES Keep only the ones you really like and add the rest to piles two and three.

BELTS These don't generally date but if you no longer have a waist and can't wear belts, they are a constant reminder of your 'waisted' days . Get rid of them or, if you are convinced that you will one day wear them, put them away in a spare wardrobe or in the loft.

JEWELLERY Go through your jewellery and evaluate it properly, particularly if you are a hoarder like me. I had earrings, a present, which made me look like Gypsy Rose Lee, as well as weird and wonderful chains from my youth that I wouldn't be seen dead in now. It's liberating to get rid of all these bits and pieces. And think what fun someone else can have with them.

UNDERWEAR Take this opportunity to go through all your drawers (no pun intended) and discard anything frayed or dingy. Get rid of the underwear you no longer wear: bras with questionable elastic, tights in obscure colours, everything and anything, in fact, that you don't wear or use.

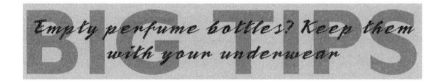

Empty perfume bottles? Keep them with your underwear

MAKE-UP Take a good look in your make-up drawer. Most women's make-up reflects the state of their wardrobe; they have a drawer full of the stuff, yet mainly select from a few favourite items. Put to one side the make-up you regularly wear. Evaluate the rest and if you haven't ever worn it, or only rarely, get rid of it. In particular, get rid of any old eye make-up. According to experts, any mascara over six months old can cause eye infections.

The Art of Wardrobe Maintenance

Now that you have sorted the wheat from the chaff in your wardrobe, the next step is to make sure you make the most of the clothes that are left. Here's your project to achieve this.

Project four — back to pile one

These are all the clothes that you do wear, that you do like and that you know you look and feel good in. Don't worry if this is only a small pile. Remember the statistic? It's probably only 15% of your wardrobe. It may even be less. This is quite normal. This important pile will be the nucleus of your new wardrobe and you need to look after it, and all your future purchases, properly.

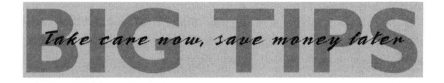

BIG TIPS

Take care now, save money later

The hanging question

All your clothes need hanging correctly so that they come out of the wardrobe in good shape and ready to wear. Here are the rules:

- **Banish wire hangers.** Return them to the dry cleaners — they don't do your clothes any favours.

- **Buy good hangers** — you can get them in any department store. You can also ask for them when you buy something; lots of stores will give you more than just one if you smile and ask politely.
- **Jackets** need hangers that are slightly wider than average and jacket-shaped — don't tell me you haven't got room for wider hangers, once you clear out the 85% of clothes you never wear, you'll have plenty of room for all your clothes to hang well.
- **Blouses** need non-slip, nicely rounded hangers.
- **There are many different styles of skirt hangers** — find one you like. *Never* hang skirts by the skirt hooks — they'll come out of the wardrobe a sloppy shape.
- **Trousers** will crease less and take up less space if you hang them by their legs.

Make sure you get good hangers in the near future. Now hang your clothes back in the wardrobe like this:

- **Hang all your jackets together**, all the skirts together, blouses together, trousers together. In other words, *don't* hang up a suit as a suit. Think of your navy suit with the matching blouse as three separate items — your navy skirt, patterned navy blouse and navy jacket. This way you will get far more use out of them than if you always think of them together as a suit.
- **Empty all your pockets** and take any brooches off your jackets before you hang them up. It's annoying when you're in a hurry and can't find your best

brooch or can't remember in which pocket you left your favourite pair of earrings.

- Do up at least the top button on jackets and blouses.
- If you have managed to get hangers that make this possible, it is useful to **hang your clothes all at the same level.**
- If you have two or more of the same thing (two blouses, for instance) in a similar colour, hang them together to **create colour categories.**
- **Divide your wardrobe into spring/summer clothes and autumn/winter clothes.** Only put back in your wardrobe the ones for the current season. Store the rest somewhere — a spare wardrobe, a suitcase, under the bed, in the loft. Stacked hangers are a good idea for putting away winter clothes in the summer or vice versa.
- **Don't leave the dry cleaning dust wraps on your clothes.** They attract dust and besides, if you can't see them, you won't wear them.
- *Never* **hang more than one garment on a hanger.** Now you have more room this won't ever be necessary.
- *Always* **hang clothes you have worn on the outside of your wardrobe overnight.** Inspect them in the morning (apart from looking for stains, give them the 'sniff' test). Put them away only if they pass with flying colours.

Wardrobe grooming kit

To make sure you can easily look after your clothes always have to hand the following:

- **Clothes brush**
- **Fluff remover**
- **Sweater comb/shaver**
- **Suede brush**
- **Bags (or special hangers) for underwear, tights, pop socks (snappy bags are ideal)**

Best foot forward

Don't forget to look after your shoes. Use shoetrees; they really do make shoes last longer. If you are a heavy person, you are probably heavy on your shoes, and you'll know that it is worth investing in good quality footwear. The more expensive the shoes, the longer you'd like them to look good. The best way to extend their life is to put shoetrees in them.

It's expensive to buy shoetrees for all your shoes, but if you buy them for your two or three most recent purchases, it's a good start. Then, each time you buy new shoes, buy another pair of shoetrees and, in a couple of years, you will have enough to last the rest of your life.

More shoe tips

- **Use Scotchguard or a similar product on new shoes** as it really does protect them and make them last longer. Always put shoes away clean.
- **Never wear the same pair of shoes two days running.** Leather is a natural fibre and needs to be allowed to breathe and recover. Leaving shoes overnight allows them to rest to a certain extent but wearing two pairs alternately will give them a much longer lease of life.

- **Put shoetrees in the shoes while they are still warm** — this stops the crease marks from solidifying.
- **Keep shoetrees in the car** so that, as you kick off those warm shoes to put on your driving shoes, the shoetrees are to hand. I put my shoetrees straight into my briefcase as I put my shoes on in the bedroom.
- **Polish shoes whilst they are warm** too as this helps the polish to sink into the leather.

If you are already doing all of the above you're a better woman than me. I can cope with the first four but the last one is too much of an effort — when I get home I'm always too busy deciding what to take out of the freezer for dinner. If you just try to make as many of them as possible a part of your routine, your shoes will appreciate the difference.

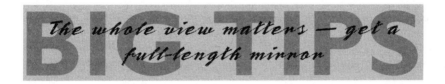

The whole view matters — get a full-length mirror

Keeping Up the Good Work

If you found projects three and four tedious, don't worry, the worst is over now. You can keep your clothes looking good in future by dealing with them swiftly just twice a year — and this is how you do it.

At the start of the spring/summer season, go through your winter clothes and put away all those that are too warm or wintry. While you're doing this, check anything you haven't worn in the past six months and, if you can see you are not going to wear it next winter, *get rid of it now.* Keep anything you feel you may wear again. If, the following year, you still have not worn that garment, then *definitely* get rid of it.

At the start of the autumn/winter season follow the same process with your summer clothes.

This should take you no more than half an hour or so twice a year and you'll never have to spend hours on a really tedious turn-out ever again.

Now each time you open your wardrobe doors you will be pleased with yourself. Your orderly wardrobe should help you to choose quickly what to wear each day, look in the mirror, and like what you see.

Wardrobe Building

Now that you've stripped your wardrobe to the core, it's time to rebuild it into one that works for you. Before I talk about your specific needs and what will suit you, the first — often neglected — step is to work out your budget.

Do you know how much you spend each year on clothes? A frightening number of women never dream of working out a budget and have no idea how much of their income they spend on themselves. Here's a statistic for you: Japanese and American women are said to spend around 33% of their income on clothes; Continental women spend 15–20% and British women 10%. So it's unlikely that you are being extravagant but, in order not to overspend and still buy enough to keep you looking good, it's only sensible to work out a budget.

Project five — know your budget

Look back at your old cheque book stubs/credit card statements/receipts and see how much you spent in the last year on clothes and accessories. Don't forget to include make-up, lingerie, tights, etc. Most people manage not to spend more than they can afford, so this will give you a good idea of your spending power — your budget.

Next, list how you spent that budget last year: how much on suits, jackets, evening wear, skirts, trousers, coats, blouses, sweaters, lingerie, tights, accessories, make-up and so on. This could be very revealing and should highlight your wise buys... and your expensive mistakes!

Wait a minute — has talk of budgeting freaked you out? Can't do it? Won't do it? Don't want to face how much you've spent?

I can sympathise. If you really can't face doing it in retrospect, please just try to keep a record over the coming year — investing some time and effort in this now will save you a lot of time and money whenever you shop in the future.

Here's a thought-provoking exercise for you: look at the examples below, then look back at some of your purchases in the last year and work out the CPW (cost per wear).

Item	Cost	Times worn in a year	Cost per wear
Suit	£200	Twice a week for nine months	£2.56
Skirt	£100	Once a week for a year	£1.92
Cashmere sweater	£100	Once a month for four months	£25
Cocktail dress	£100	Once	£100

BIG TIPS
Budgeting is good for you

Interesting, isn't it? When you look at it like this, you can easily see that what appeared at the time to be an expensive purchase was worth every penny, while the cashmere sweater, even though it was half price in the sales, was not a true bargain. It's so easy to spend a lot of money on an eye-catching item that you can only wear occasionally, when it's much better value to spend that money on something you will wear frequently.

We have now come full circle from the beginning of this chapter — have you spent most of your money where you spend most of your time? If not, I hope you now have a clearer idea of what this means and can resolve to do better in the future.

Identify the Gaps

Now that you know what's in your wardrobe and how much you've got to spend, you can identify what's missing; and therefore what you need to buy to create a comprehensive collection of clothes for your lifestyle. Are you a casual dresser with only one pair of jeans? Or a businesswoman with a serious shortage of suits? Try drawing up a list of clothes you really need.

Basic business wardrobe
- SUITS If you wear a suit every day, you need a
  minimum of three — two neutral (find out what this
  means in Chapter Six) and one patterned, which will

mix and match. Wear them in rotation — they will last longer as the fabric gets a chance to rest and breathe.

- JACKETS At least two — in your best neutrals.
- SKIRTS A minimum of three, to match or blend with your jackets and the jackets from your suits.
- TROUSERS If these are acceptable for your work, you need at least one pair, preferably two, to match or blend with your jackets and turn them into trouser suits.
- BLOUSES A minimum of ten, two white, the others plain or patterned.
- COAT Coat and/or raincoat in a neutral tones (see Chapter Six again).
- SHOES A minimum of three pairs.
- BELTS Two or three good quality leather belts. (Only if you have a waist.) See more about belts on page 148.
- ACCESSORIES Always buy the very best you can afford.

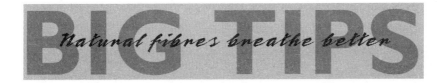

BIG TIPS

Natural fibres breathe better

A casual approach

Perhaps it is quite acceptable for you to dress casually for work. Or perhaps you work from home and nobody but the cat ever sees you. Or you could be at home all day with the children. I still suggest you aim for a casual/smart look rather than a casual/slobby look — it's far better for your morale and you'll work better, talk on the 'phone with more authority and feel better about yourself in relation to your children because you are taking care of your appearance. Ensure that your hair is neat and tidy and try a little lipstick and mascara to make you feel good about yourself.

Foundations Matter

You'll only look your best on the outside if what you've got on underneath provides a good base to build on. The right underwear is crucial to how you look and how comfortable you feel, and it's worth taking a little time over. In contrast, here's how not to do it.

Angela Giveon, Editor of the quarterly magazine *Executive Woman*, tells how she had a date to attend an extremely swish function with a very desirable man. The outfit she planned to wear was slightly too small and made her feel like the Michelin man, so she splashed out on an all-in-one corselette — two sizes too small.

Unfortunately, during dinner, she began to feel as if the garment was trying to cut her in two. The wonderful man wanted to dance but that was out of the question, she could barely walk. Finally, she took herself off to the cloakroom and found that being cut in half wasn't just a metaphor — the corset literally had cut her skin. She broke four nails trying to scrabble out of the garment, without success, and the cloakroom attendant eventually had to cut her out — causing the whole thing to roll up like a shutter. She had to keep the corset on because she needed the bra for support but it was now such hell to sit down that she made her bewildered date dance the rest of the night away.

Bras

There are many so-called bosom exercises, but breast tissue is not muscle. Once stretched, it cannot be toned and no amount of Jane Fonda-ing will get it back in shape. I cannot over-emphasise the importance of wearing a good bra that fits you well. A large bosom needs the correct size bra to ensure it looks smaller and firmer — this is an engineering weight-distribution exercise! Incidentally, if you have a heavy bust and want a dress which requires a strapless bra, be warned — very few come in large cup sizes. Before you spend money on the dress, make sure you can find the appropriate bra. Here are a few tips on ensuring you wear the right size in any kind of bra. (My thanks to Margaret Ann for her contribution to this section.)

● **There are many ways of being measured but none as accurate as having an expert do it for you.** Your bra size is a combination of your underbust measurement (called the back size) and your around-the-bosom measurement (called the cup size). When were you last expertly measured for a bra? You should have it done annually. It's amazing how your size can change even if your weight never fluctuates.

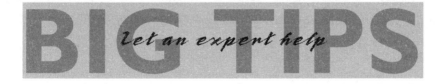

● **A new bra should be done up on the middle row of the three rows of hooks.** Then, if you are pre-menstrual, you can loosen it, and when it has been well worn and is losing its elasticity, it can be done up on the tightest row.

- **If your bra is too tight on the loosest set of hooks,** you need a larger size. Similarly, **if it is most comfortable done up on the tightest set,** a new bra is a must. And each time you buy a bra, be measured for it, as your figure changes with any weight fluctuations.

- **If the back of your bra rides up you need a smaller back size.** As with clothes, each manufacturer makes to a slightly different specification so if you buy a bra from a different manufacturer, it won't automatically be in the same size as one you already possess. Fit is also affected by different cups and fabrics. If you need a 44 DD in one style, in another you may need a 42 E. Generally speaking, if you go down a back size, then you need to go up a cup size.

- **If your bosom is slightly bulging over the top or sides of your bra,** you need one cup size larger. If it's bulging more than this, you may need two or three cup sizes larger, or a larger back size too.

- **If you have a large, heavy bust you should avoid narrow straps and backs.** Basically, if you find that the straps of your bra are cutting in, the whole bra, and in particular the cups, are too small.

Nursing bras

- **A pre-natal bra is as important as a nursing bra** and this is a much neglected area. This needs to be a soft bra, purchased as soon as you realise you are pregnant. A soft bra allows breast growth as pregnancy develops — a wired bra restricts the growth of the breast and the development of the milk ducts.

- **Nursing bras should be fitted six weeks before the baby is due.**
- There should be a gap over the nipple area to allow for growth and room for breast pads when the milk comes in. **A good nursing bra will have four sets of hooks on the back to allow for support and, when the milk comes in, plenty of latitude for growth.** It must never be too tight as this can cause mastitis. Drop cups and zip cups are available, but do be careful if you zip or unzip in a hurry — *ouch!*

Pants

From thongs and G-strings to cami-knickers, there's a huge choice in pants, but I advise larger women to stick to full briefs, which comfortably cover your whole bottom. They may not be the sexiest things around, but there's nothing worse than knickers that ride up your bottom, or which your bottom visibly bulges out of, or clothes which are so tight that your panty-line shows. Control pants can be a good idea, but be warned, pantie girdles, or anything firmer, just tend to push the excess flab somewhere else.

Bodies

I constantly hear clients and friends praising the comforts of bodysuits, but until recently I could never find one in my size.

If you hanker after one, too, you will find that they are available in larger sizes in mail-order catalogues.

If you are built like me, however, you may find them a bit of a challenge to put on.

I was trying my new body on and as I bent down to fasten it, the rear flap flipped up out of reach. I tried to reach it several times with no success, simply causing paroxyms of laughter in my husband. After calming him down enough to grab the flap for me, I bent down to do up the press studs, only to find that my boobs were in the way and I couldn't see at the right angle through my variofocal lenses anyway. I gave up, but tried again next day (alone!) and succeeded after about 15 minutes; but I have to say that the idea of being stuck in this predicament in the loo during a business meeting put me off rather, and I sent the body back for a refund.

Don't let my experience put you off, though. If you fancy one, give it a go.

Hosiery

Most large women prefer tights to stockings as they look more streamlined. An essential for me, when wearing tights on a hot day, is also to wear a cotton culotte slip. It's actually cooler to wear this extra layer and it stops chafing between the legs. Control-topped tights can give welcome support for your stomach, but never wear them one size too small as they can force your stomach up over the waistband, creating unsightly bulges.

Plea to manufacturers: do you realise how many women (small as well as large, if my clients are anything to go by) have difficulty finding tights that are the right size all round? Could we have labels in the waistbands — instead of on the wrappings — so we can remember which ones fitted best when we come to buy some more?

Swimsuits

If you are 5ft 6in or over, don't automatically dismiss a two-piece swimsuit. A long line bottom and good boned bra can look extremely good. Otherwise, a one-piece is your best bet (see more tips on swimsuits on pages 118–19).

Suitcase Surgery

This is a bit of an aside, but it's useful to know that the tactics you used on your wardrobe can also be applied to packing your suitcase for a holiday or business trip. Do you always pack too much? Do all those 'just-in-case' items mean you need an extra suitcase? Once you've reorganised your wardrobe and have fewer clothes to choose from it will be so much easier.

With a bit of forethought, taking less makes for much easier packing and unpacking. And if you take clothes that mix and match you actually take less but have more to wear!

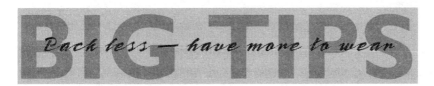

BIG TIPS

Pack less — have more to wear

Ten top travel tips
- **Pack to suit the climate you're going to.** If it's going to be variable, take clothes that you can layer, plus thermal underwear, rather than bulky sweaters.

- **Do you really need something totally different for each day?** Even if you see the same people every day, they won't notice if you wear the same thing more than once, particularly if you team it up with something different each time.
- **First decide which neutral colour** (see Chapter Six) **you will base your packing around.** Then select only the clothes that can be worn with this neutral. This immediately eliminates the need for a specific pair of shoes and matching handbag to wear with just one outfit.
- **You'll probably need at least three pairs of shoes, even if they are all the same colour:** flatties for walking, sandals for casual (or classic court shoes if you are on business) and smarter shoes for evening. Two handbags should be sufficient, one for day, another for evening. If you need a briefcase, make the evening bag a clutch bag, then it will fit in the briefcase and double as a purse for lunchtime.
- On a business trip, **skirts and jackets will give you more mix-and-match choices than suits.**
- A few days before packing hang up all the clothes you plan to take on the outside of a wardrobe and really evaluate your choice. Choose shoes and handbags to complement your outfits. Select scarves, jewellery, belts, hosiery etc., to go with your clothes. *Never take anything that does not go with at least two other items.*
- **Check that everything is spotless,** buttons firmly attached, hems in place, shoes heeled and cleaned.

- **Pack as hand luggage all that you will need for the first thirty-six hours of your trip, in case your baggage goes astray.** The larger you are the more essential this is — it's hard enough to buy clothes quickly on familiar territory; doing it when newly-arrived in a foreign country is my idea of a nightmare.
- **Check that your hotel has good laundry facilities and a hairdryer** or take Travel Wash, a travelling iron and your own hairdryer (remember to check plugs and the strength of the current).
- **Hang up your clothes on arrival.** If anything is heavily creased, hang it in the bathroom and run a hot bath or shower — the steam will help the creases drop out.

Successful Shopping

You should now be very aware of:

- **What is in your wardrobe**
- **Your budget**
- **What you actually need to buy**

The next step is shopping. This can be a dispiriting experience for many large women. The next three chapters will give you lots of help in identifying what shapes and colours to look for so your shopping expeditions will be more rewarding, but first there are a few basic rules:

- **Allow plenty of time.** This may sound like a joke for the busy working woman or those with children,

but just think of the mistakes you've made when
you've shopped in a hurry. Organise your outing so
that you *do* have the time.

- **Dress appropriately.** You really can't tell if a skirt
  is the right length if you're wearing socks and
  sneakers. Besides, if you're well dressed you'll get
  better attention from shop assistants.
- Most important of all, **do not buy anything unless
  it goes with *at least* two, preferably three,
  other items in your wardrobe.**

The Perfect Fit

Another fundamental shopping rule is to make sure that
everything you buy fits. That's obvious, I hear you say, but it's
amazing how many women don't take the time to check this
properly. You're shopping in a hurry, the changing room is
crowded, you're trying a jacket with just a T-shirt on
underneath: for all these reasons, you may find that the
garment that seemed so perfect in the shop doesn't look
right after all. Follow these guidelines for a really good fit.

Jackets
- **Even if you never do up a jacket, make sure
  that it is possible to do it up.** If you can't fasten it
  with ease, it doesn't fit properly across your
  shoulders and bust.
- **Always allow that little bit extra,** too, just in
  case you want to wear a sweater underneath.
- **The sleeve of a classic jacket should touch the
  wristbone.**

TAKING THE PLUNGE 77

Coats and macs

When trying on either of these, make sure that there is room for a jacket underneath, particularly if you're shopping on a hot day when jackets are furthest from your mind. If you don't have one with you, borrow one from another department in the shop or store.

Skirts

- **Skirts should be loose enough to turn around your body easily and to ensure that your panty line doesn't show.**
- **You should be able to insert two fingers widthways into the waistband.**

Trousers

- **Trousers need to hang from your hip,** not curve under your bottom or show your panty line.
- As with a skirt, **use the two-fingers-widthways-in-the-waistband test.**

Blouses

- **Blouses must *not* pull at the bust.**
- **With a jacket over the top, the blouse sleeve should be about a quarter of an inch longer than the jacket sleeve.**

I cannot emphasize enough the importance of wearing clothes that are not too tight. Many large women kid themselves about their size and squeeze into clothes one, or even two sizes too small. Apart from being uncomfortable, this emphasizes every lump and bump. The label in the garment is irrelevant. This is not just a neurosis of large women. I've had size 12 clients who've needed a size 14 in some garment, but simply will not buy it because the label says 14 and she's adamant that she's a 12. If you try something on that says it's your size and it's too big, you're only too happy to go down a size or two. Please, do the opposite, too, disregard the label and buy the size that flatters you most.

Have Fun

Finally, and importantly, make sure you have lots of fun when you shop. Never go out with a set item in mind, like a red blouse or a green skirt. You can bet your bottom dollar you won't find one you like in the right size or in a shade that you like and you'll come home empty-handed. How depressing!

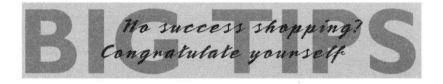

BIG TIPS

No success shopping?
Congratulate yourself

The answer is to make sure this never happens. If you don't find any clothes that are right, treat yourself to a little something that will bring a smile to your face as you put the kettle on. Perhaps your favourite magazine, a new CD, a pair of earrings — for me it would be a bunch of freesias — and *congratulate yourself* ... you haven't wasted any money which means you'll have more to spend when you do find the right thing.

If you see something you like — it's a good colour and a flattering style — buy it, even if you don't know when you'll wear it. It will be hanging there in your wardrobe just waiting for the right occasion. And if the occasion never materialises, wear it anyway — you already know you'll feel good and look great in it.

Making Progress

Follow my guidelines and you will quickly achieve a well co-ordinated and extremely manageable wardrobe. Your aim is never to shop in a panic again, as you'll always have something suitable to wear.

Now you know how to do it in principle, but you still may not be sure which are the best colours and styles for you. That's what comes next, so arm yourself by reading the following chapters, then go out and shop with confidence.

CHAPTER FOUR

Face Facts

'YOUR FACE IS YOUR COMMUNICATION CENTRE'

I've already mentioned the importance of eye contact. One of the best ways to establish — and keep — eye contact is to frame your face attractively. It's the focus of all your direct contact with other people — your communication centre — so make sure it gets the attention it deserves. When it comes to faces, large women often have an advantage over their slimmer friends. Many have better, firmer skin and fewer 'laugh lines' — a bonus from that extra layer of fat.

I'm going to begin looking at style in this book by talking about face shapes. You might have thought that body shapes would come first, but to really get your style spot-on, you first need to know your face shape and learn to frame it in the most complimentary way you can. The frame you'll be looking at is the area from your shoulders upwards.

Lines can either be straight or curved. Starting at the basics, you need to establish whether your face is angular, with a bone structure that forms straight lines; or contoured (curvy), with a bone structure that forms curving lines: this affects everything else — your choice of hairstyles, jewellery, glasses, necklines and hats.

There are eight basic face shapes:

Oval

The lines of your face curve and taper gently from forehead to chin. Your forehead is slightly wider than your chin — think of an egg. You probably have high cheekbones and you'll be pleased to know that this shape is always referred to in beauty books as the 'perfect' face shape because it appears to be nicely balanced and in proportion. The length of your face is greater than the width.

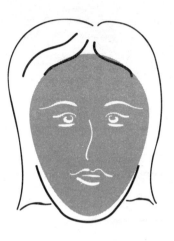

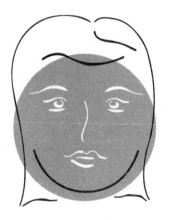

Round

Your face looks full with few angles — this is a very symmetrical shape. Your cheeks are the widest part and the lines of your face are curved, including a rounded hairline and chin. The length and width of your face appear roughly equal.

Heart/Inverted Triangle

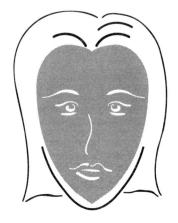 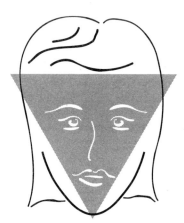

You have high cheekbones and your forehead is the widest part of your face, tapering to a narrow jaw. If the bone structure and lines are quite straight, you're a triangle (inverted), an angular shape. But if the lines curve gently, you're a heart.

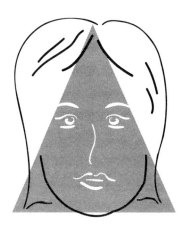

Pear/Triangle

You have a narrow forehead that gradually becomes wider at the cheek and chin areas. If your bone structure is quite straight, you have a triangular face, but if its lines curve gently, then your face is pear-shaped.

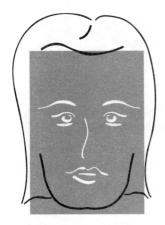

Oblong

You have a long face, with fairly straight lines, though they may curve gently. Your forehead, cheeks and jawline are similar in width, although your cheeks may be slightly wider. The length of your face is noticeably greater than the width.

Square

The lines of your face are straight and you have a square, broad jawline. Your hairline is straight and you have a wide forehead, too — this is again a symmetrical shape. The length and width of your face may seem pretty equal, or the length can be slightly greater than the width.

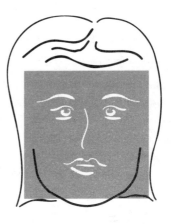

Diamond

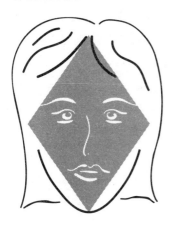

You have a small forehead, widening at the cheekbones and eye area and then gradually tapering to a small chin. Most women with this face shape naturally choose a hairstyle to disguise their small forehead, which turns their face into an inverted triangle The lines of your face are quite straight.

A summary

- **Oval, round, pear and heart-shaped faces are contoured.** Look at all those curves.
- **Oblong, square, diamond and triangle-shaped faces are angular.** Follow the straight lines along the outline.

Analyse Your Face Shape

Here's how to assess whether your face is angular or contoured.

Sit in front of a mirror, pin your hair back off your face and study your bone structure. Do you see angles (straight lines) or contours (curves)? Don't pay attention to any extra flesh there is around, if necessary push it gently out of the way with the flat of your hand to reveal the underlying bone structure.

If you still can't decide which you are, don't worry. Try this trick. Put on a T-shirt with a high, round neck. *Really* look hard at yourself. Now pull that neckline down to create a 'V'. Which looks best? Does one neckline make your face look slimmer? If you decide the round neckline looks best, your face is one of the contoured shapes. If the 'V' neck is better, then your face is one of the angular shapes.

Still not sure? See if you can find two similar-sized (not dangly) earrings, one round, the other oblong. Put one on each ear. Hide one ear and examine your features. Now hide the other ear and look again. If your face looks best with the oblong earring, you have an angular face shape. If the round earring does you more favours, you have a contoured face shape.

Hair — Shapes and Styles

It's important to choose a hairstyle that flatters your face shape. Here are some general guidelines:

OVAL Good news! Most hairstyles will suit you.

ROUND You need a soft hairstyle. If your kind of hair allows, bring some of it on to the sides of your face to disguise the width. Add height to your hairstyle, with a perm perhaps, to help balance your head with the rest of your body.

HEART Your face needs fullness at chin level to help balance your broad forehead. An off-centre parting will help soften that forehead, too.

PEAR Your face needs a soft hairstyle, kept away from your jawline, with fullness on the forehead to balance the fullness of your cheeks.

TRIANGLE/INVERTED TRIANGLE The same advice applies as for heart and pear shapes, but create an angular rather than a soft style.

OBLONG An asymmetrical hairstyle will emphasise and flatter angles. An off-centre parting works well, too. If you have a particularly long face, don't add height — but try a fringe, it'll shorten your face and make it look more balanced. Long, straight hair is out, it will just elongate your features. If you have a slim oblong face then fullness at the sides will look good. If you have a full oblong face, keep the sides flatter and your face will look slimmer.

SQUARE If you can add height to your hairstyle, it'll lengthen your face. An asymmetrical style will do good things to the angles in your face.

DIAMOND If you don't have one already, experiment with a fringe to add fullness at your forehead. An angular style will emphasise those cheekbones.

General tips

- Logically enough, **if your face shape is contoured,** a soft, curvy, symmetrical hairstyle will frame your features best.
- **For an angular face shape,** you're better off with an asymmetrical, more angular hairstyle.
- **Like a perm?** With an angular face shape, try a soft body wave rather than corkscrew curls. If your face is contoured, you're lucky, you can take a tight perm or a soft body wave.
- **Prefer to keep your hair short?** Whatever your face shape, keep the hair behind the ears just that little bit longer, so it shows from the front. Otherwise, if you have a large body, your head can look like a pimple on St. Paul's (Cathedral!). If you have a short neck or a double chin, a bit of length behind the ears is more flattering than a really short style.

Baubles and Bangles

The size of the jewellery you wear should generally relate to your height and your body size. As a basic guideline:

- **If you are under 5ft 1in your jewellery needs to be small to medium sized.**
- **If you are 5ft 2in–5ft 6in your jewellery needs to be medium to large**

- **If you are 5ft 7in and over your jewellery needs to be large to overscale**

However, here's a story that shows that you shouldn't stick rigidly to rules.

Rachel is a size 20 and 5ft 1in. She has a big, round face, huge eyes, a generous mouth and wide smile. Someone once told her that, as she has a petite frame, she should wear small earrings — what nonsense! When I met her she was wearing tiny pearl studs — lovely earrings, and perfect if she were a short woman with a quiet personality. But Rachel, with her bouncy, vibrant, dramatic personality, can carry much larger, more extrovert earrings — the tiny ones were totally out of keeping.

I'm going to outline some general advice on which earrings are likely to suit your face shape best, but don't see it as a straitjacket. Some earrings can have elements of the 'wrong' style for you and still be flattering — go by what you see in the mirror; and if your favourite earrings, a cherished gift perhaps, are completely the 'wrong' shape, there's no need to give up wearing them, as long as they make you feel good and you try to counterbalance them with other elements that are right for you.

Choosing earrings

As you would expect, women with contoured face shapes should look for jewellery with curvy lines, while geometric, angular jewellery is for women with angular faces. Here are a few more details of what to look out for.

OVAL FACE You fortunate, oval-faced women will find most earrings suit you. But be careful of very long shapes — they will elongate your features and spoil that 'perfect' balance.

ROUND FACE In theory, round earrings should be your best style, but if you have a full, round face, they will exaggerate it. Try ovals — they should elongate and balance your features.

HEART/INVERTED TRIANGLE/DIAMOND FACE Look for earrings with width at the bottom to offset your narrow chin.

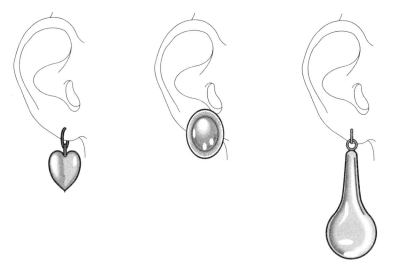

Here are sample earrings to suit some (l. to r.) oval, round and inverted triangle or diamond-shaped faces. Remember that what will actually suit you will depend on your own taste and personality.

PEAR/TRIANGLE FACE It's best to avoid earrings which finish level with your jawline as this will only make it look wider — go for upswept styles.

OBLONG FACE Oblong or square earrings are for you. If you have a very long face, go for wider earrings, they'll add width and make your face seem shorter. Give ovals a try, too — you'll find they work surprisingly well.

SQUARE FACE For square faces, an oblong, or softened oblong, is the most flattering, as they will visually soften and lengthen your face.

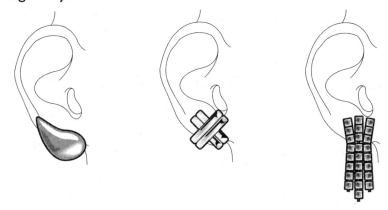

These examples would suit some (l. to r.) square, oblong and inverted triangle or diamond face shapes.

Clients often ask my advice on wearing long, dangly earrings. If you'd like to, but aren't sure if they'd suit you, look at yourself in the mirror. Where does the bottom of your earlobe come to? Is it in line with your bottom lip, or with the tip of your nose, or higher on your face? The higher your ears are set on your face, the more likely it is that long earrings will suit you. Be warned, though, they're best avoided if you have a short neck or a double chin. Even if you decide they do suit you, it can be better to keep dangly earrings for the evening. They may not be appropriate in all work environments.

Choosing necklaces

The same sort of guidelines apply to necklaces as to earrings. Geometric shapes suit the angular faces and rounded shapes suit the contoured faces.

Tips

- If you have a **round face, a short neck or double chin,** avoid choker-style necklaces, as these make your face look rounder and your neck look shorter.
- **Long necklaces elongate the neck and face** (though if you have a large chest, be careful that necklaces don't dangle 'over the edge'; stick to medium-length necklaces that sit on top of your bosom).
- Don't wear a necklace *and* a brooch and earrings. A necklace should match or complement *either* earrings or a brooch.

Necklines

By this point I'm sure you are beginning to get the feel of what you should be looking for to frame your face.

Necklines for contoured features are: jewel, rounded, scooped, short cowl, crew and turtleneck, ruffled, draped and any shape that has a curved finish, such as bows at the neck and collars with rounded corners or a curved mandarin.

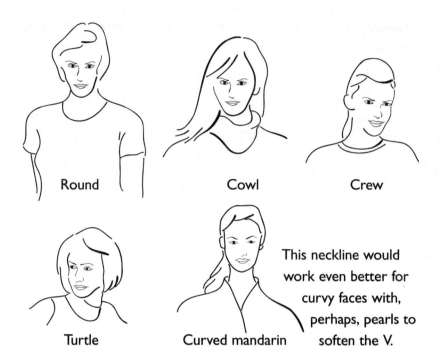

Round

Cowl

Crew

Turtle

Curved mandarin

This neckline would work even better for curvy faces with, perhaps, pearls to soften the V.

Lapels that suit contoured features best are shawl collars, rounded collars and softly notched lapels — any style that has a soft, curvy look.

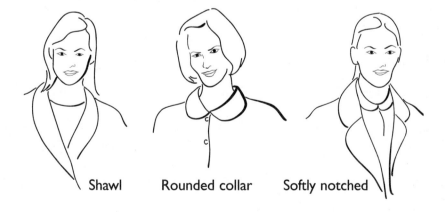

Shawl

Rounded collar

Softly notched

Necklines to flatter an angular face are square, V-shaped, long cowl, crisp mandarin and any shape that has crisp, clean lines, such as collars with pointed corners.

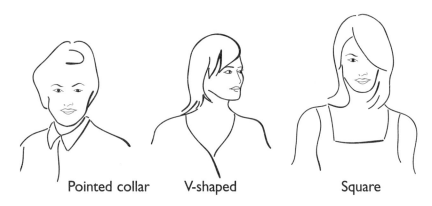

Pointed collar   V-shaped   Square

Lapels will enhance your angular features best if they are notched and have a sharp, angular look.

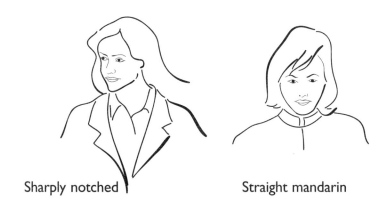

Sharply notched   Straight mandarin

Low necklines will suit most face shapes, and so do sweetheart, scooped, boatneck and polo necklines.

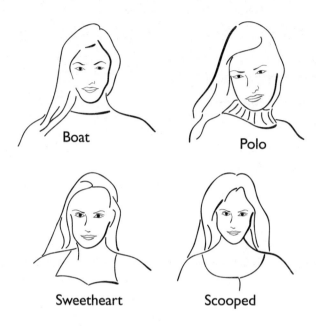

Boat   Polo

Sweetheart   Scooped

Keep it in Perspective

I hope you'll find the information above useful, but *please* don't drive yourself crazy with it. Just be aware of the optimum look for your features so that if ever you have anything made you will know precisely what you want.

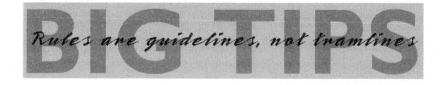

BIG TIPS

Rules are guidelines, not tramlines

Meanwhile, if you see something in the shops that is a good colour and style for you (you'll find out more about these aspects in the following chapters), and it's a price that you like, for goodness' sake, buy it. If the neckline is not ideal for your features, you can make it work by wearing earrings plus a necklace or brooch that *are* right to balance the effect.

In other words, listen to the rules, but learn how to bend them successfully.

Tips for double chins
- *Don't* wear choker-style necklaces, polo or turtle necks, mandarin collars, buttoned-up collars, high-tied scarves. If you like the warmth of a polo neck, however, wear a V-necked sweater over the top or a long necklace that falls in a V to give the illusion of a longer neck.
- *Do* wear scoop and V-necks, long necklaces, open collars, loosely tied scarves.

Go Ahead, Get a Hat

Do you hate wearing a hat? You are not alone. From what I hear, most women feel very self-conscious in a hat. There are a fortunate few who have realised that it gives them extra poise and makes them stand out in a crowd, but they are in the minority.

If there's an occasion when you *must* wear a hat, learn how to choose the right one for your features and to feel more comfortable with it on.

Top ten hat tips
- Usually, when you try on a hat, it's in front of a mirror which only shows your head and shoulders. Once you think you have selected a hat you like,

find a full-length mirror (it shouldn't be too hard in a department store, or other clothes shop) and have a good look to make sure that it's in proportion with the rest of you.

- **The brim** should be no wider than your shoulders and the crown should be as wide as the widest part of your face.
- **If you are short, but fancy wearing a big hat** (though you've read that you shouldn't), look for one that is made from transparent material and you'll look great!
- **Buy your outfit *first*,** then look for a matching or contrasting hat. Take your outfit or at least part of your outfit — perhaps the jacket — with you to make absolutely sure that not only is the hat the right colour but also the right style for the outfit. You simply cannot do this from memory.
- As always, **a contoured face shape requires a hat with curvy lines, perhaps with a curved brim or a rounded crown.** Don't wear it at too much of an angle, it'll clash with the curves.
- Likewise, an angular face shape likes a hat that has a more angular look to it. **Top tip:** even a hat that looks quite curvy will look more angular worn at a rakish angle. If you need a hat pin, look for angular decoration.

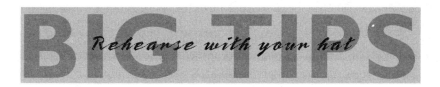

BIG TIPS
Rehearse with your hat

- **Hat pins are fun,** and essential for certain styles and windy days. Use one to enhance your contoured face — look for a pin with a curved decoration.
- **Don't expect to put on a hat and magically look and feel special.** First of all, it must be comfortable. If it's too tight, you'll end up with a headache; too loose, and it could end up in a puddle. Find one that feels just right and, if you want security, anchor it with hat pins or elastic under your hair — or both. The elastic is meant to be worn beneath the hair at the nape of your neck and this may not be enough to keep it on in a strong wind. If a hat pin is not suitable, use some hidden pins.
- **Formal hats** usually look best with as little hair as possible showing. Wear long hair up and out of the way.
- If you are not used to wearing a hat, it can completely mar your enjoyment of a special occasion, so don't wear it for the first time on the day, **make sure you have a dress rehearsal beforehand.** Wait till all the family are out. Take your ironing board into your bedroom or wherever you have a full-length mirror. Pour yourself a glass of wine — you're probably going to need it — and iron for at least one hour, *wearing the hat.* Talk to yourself in the mirror, chat with some fictitious guests, sip your wine and *enjoy.* By the end of an hour the hat won't feel strange on your head and, when you wear it for the function, it will feel like an old friend.
- **Either wear an eye-catching hat and a plain outfit or an eye-catching outfit and a plain hat** — *NEVER BOTH AT THE SAME TIME.*

Specs Appeal

If you wear glasses, there is no quicker way to transform your look than by changing them. And you can dramatically enhance your facial features by choosing the right colour and style of frames.

For many women, eyewear has evolved from a pure necessity to a high-powered fashion accessory. By simply changing your glasses you can go from classic to chic, refined to fun-loving, serious to glamorous.

Glasses are a far more important and visible accessory than your handbag, yet many women have only one pair. It is certainly quite an expense to have several pairs. To put it in perspective I often ask a female client whether she would use the same handbag to go out in the evening as to go to the supermarket in the morning. Enough said? Likewise, you'll really benefit from more than one pair of glasses. Worried about the cost? Look at it this way: if your glasses (frames and lenses) cost you £250 and you wear them every day, and change them every three years, they cost you twenty-three pence per day. On that basis, if you buy a new pair each year for three years and wear them all the same amount, then having three pairs will cost you sixty-nine pence per day — not much really, is it? And you'll feel the benefit of being able to ring the changes according to your mood, your work and your destination for that day. Treat yourself to a new pair of glasses each year and you will always have at least three on the go at any one time.

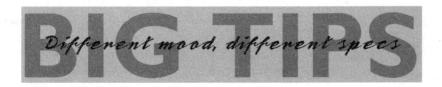

BIG TIPS

Different mood, different specs

Three pairs of glasses can complement your whole wardrobe. Get specs to co-ordinate with all your work outfits to make you feel confident and competent, a sporty pair for the weekend and a sophisticated pair for evenings out.

The colour of your frames should reflect your personal colouring. In Chapter Six you will learn whether you are 'warm' or 'cool' and whether you look better in deep or light colours, or bright, vibrant colours or soft, muted tones. When the clothes in your wardrobe reflect your colouring, your glasses should tone in with them. The shape of the frames is equally important, though, and that's what I have something to say about here.

Frames for faces

OVAL Most styles look good on an oval face. The best are frames which will not break the natural balance of your face and features:

- **Frames** that follow the natural lines of your face and are in proportion to its size.
- **Styles** the same width as, or slightly wider than, your cheeks.
- **Avoid** low or upswept sides as this will disturb the oval balance of your face.
- **If your weight is making your face look nearly round, follow the advice for a round face shape.**

ROUND You need to choose frames which will make your face appear longer as this will slim it down:

- **Angular styles, with softened edges** — not round but not too angular. Avoid round or square styles unless you want to make a statement about your round face.
- **Frames** with sides positioned mid to high, to create the illusion of a more oval face shape.
- **A clear bridge** will also give the illusion of narrowing your face, making it look more oval.
- **Frames with colour on the vertical sides** also make your face longer.
- **Avoid** decorative side pieces as this will only accentuate the width of your face.

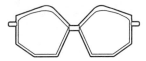

HEART/INVERTED TRIANGLE You need to look for frames which will add width to your chin and cheeks and make your forehead appear less wide:

- **Frames which are no wider than your forehead at the top, becoming wider at the bottom.**
- **Frames which are rounded at the top and squared at the bottom.**
- Either **angular or slightly curved frames.**
- **A rectangular frame** would be an excellent choice as it will make your jawline appear wider.

- **Frames with more colour on the lower half** would balance your face and add width to your jaw.
- **Low sides** also add balance to this face shape.

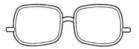

PEAR/TRIANGLE You need to look for frames which will soften your jawline and make it appear less wide, and frames which will give the illusion of a wider forehead:

- **Frames as wide as, but no wider than, your jawline,** which increase in width at the top — this will visually widen your forehead and balance your face well.
- A good choice would be **wire frames with rimless bottoms — a rectangular shape would also work very well for you.**
- **Frames which look heavier on the top than the bottom** will create good balance.
- **Avoid low side pieces** as this will add weight to your jawline — side pieces high on the frame are your optimum.

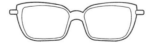

OBLONG If your face is very long, you need to choose frames which will make it look wider and shorter:

- **Frames that are wider than the widest part of your face.**
- **Deep frames or square frames** with rounded edges (or squared-off, round frames) will shorten and soften your face shape.
- **Interesting or contrasting side pieces** will add width to your face.
- **Low side pieces and low bridges** will also give your face a shorter, more oval look.
- A style with **coloured horizontal lines** will shorten this face shape. However, if your face is only just an oblong and quite plump, look for coloured vertical lines as they will visually lengthen and slim your face.

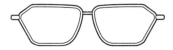

SQUARE You need to select frames that will narrow and lengthen your face:

- **Frames with softly curved styles, the same width or no wider than the widest part of your face.**
- **Slightly angular styles with curved corners** are better than completely angular styles.
- **Frames with more colour or weight at the top** will add length. So will colour on the vertical sides of frames.
- **Frames with depth rather than width** will add length to your face.

- **High side pieces** will make your face look longer. Look for unusual or interesting contrast to the side pieces as this will also help to balance your face.

DIAMOND You need to look for frames which will add width to your forehead and jawline:

- **Softly curved frames, square frames or frames which are straight at the top and rounded at the bottom.** Your frames should be no wider than the widest part of your face — your cheekbones.
- **Frames which are wider at the bottom** to balance your narrow chin.
- **Avoid decorative side pieces** as this will make your face look wider and off-balance.

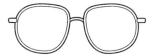

More specs tips
- **If you have a long nose,** make the middle section of your face look shorter with a frame that has a low or a clear bridge.
- **If you have a short nose,** make it look longer by choosing a keyhole bridge or a high bridge.

- **If you have a wide nose,** a dark-toned bridge that sits close to the nose will seem to slim it down. Nose pads, if you find them comfortable, will also give the illusion of a slimmer nose.
- **If you have close-set eyes,** frames with a clear bridge graduating to darker colours at the temples will make them appear wider (you probably already use this technique in the way you apply your eyeshadow).
- **If you have wide-set eyes,** a dark-coloured bridge will quite dramatically make your eyes appear closer-set.

You should now be ready to go out, armed with all this advice, to choose some wonderful new frames. You can discuss in detail with your optician the best styles and colours to suit your own colouring and features. The optician will be able to advise you on the practicality of the style you choose in relation to your particular prescription.

From Faces to Bodies

I hope you now feel more aware of your face shape, and know what suits you from your shoulders upwards. Have fun comparing and experimenting with the different necklines and accessories — you'll really see the difference they can make and learn what to look for when you buy new things.

Similar guidelines apply to body shapes, and that's what we're moving on to next.

CHAPTER FIVE

The Body in Question

'YOU WOULDN'T PUT A ROUND TABLECLOTH ON A SQUARE TABLE SO WHY PUT CURVY CLOTHES ON A STRAIGHT BODY'

*W*hen you go clothes shopping has it ever occurred to you to think about your body shape when you look at something on its hanger, before you even consider trying it on? Don't fret, nor do most women. This chapter is going to help you identify your body shape so, as with your face, you know where you have curvy (contoured) lines and where you have straight (angular) lines. When you know your own body line, you will be able to see at a glance whether something is likely to suit you and not waste time trying on things that won't.

Shopaholic or Shopaphobic?

First, though, it's worth acknowledging your attitude to shopping. A shopaholic loves it; a shopaphobic avoids it like the plague. You probably know which you are: a shopaholic spends spare cash as soon as she has any, could spend all day shopping and come home exhausted, but happy, buys things even if she's not sure she needs them, as long as she thinks they'll go with something in her wardrobe and generally enjoys the whole shopping experience. A shopaphobic only goes shopping if she really has to, and does what's necessary as quickly as possible, often buys things she doesn't like when she gets home and generally feels she looks awful in anything she buys, so what's the point?

Whichever you are, knowing your body shape will help you with your shopping. If you're a shopaphobic, it will help you shop quickly and effectively. You'll be able to get the once-hated shopping trips over and done with much more quickly.

If you love shopping, being confident of what suits your body shape will make shopping the pleasure that it should be.

The Secret of Success

Before your next shopping expedition, find out by reading this chapter whether your body has curvy or straight lines. Taken in conjunction with your face shape, it will tell you which clothes will suit you best. If your face and body are curvy then, you've guessed it, curves in all your clothes and accessories will be best for you. If your face and body both have straight lines, then straighter lines in what you wear will do the most for you.

Many people are a mixture of straight and curvy lines. In this case, you will look and feel better if you put straight lines where your body or face is straight and curvy lines where you are curvy. Simple, isn't it?

What's Your Shape?

I'm going to keep this exercise as simple as possible by referring to only four main body shapes. You should be able to fit yourself into one of these categories. Look at the pictures and decide which shape is most like you:

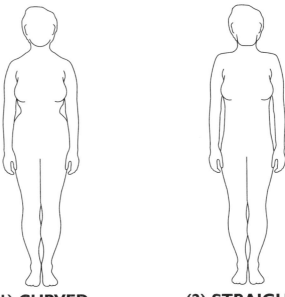

(1) CURVED	(2) STRAIGHT
Curvy face, curvy body	**Straight face, straight body**

Take a critical look at yourself. Just because you're large does not necessarily mean you're curvy. Likewise, just because your waist has disappeared doesn't mean you have a straight body. Despite any extra weight, your basic bone structure

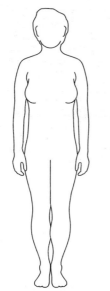

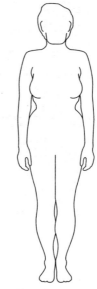

(3) SOFT/STRAIGHT   **(4) STRAIGHT/SOFT**

Curvy face, straight body   **Straight face, curvy body**

won't have changed. The best way to study your bone structure is to put on something tight-fitting, for example a pair of thick tights or leggings, with a leotard or swimming costume on top. If you don't possess a leotard or swimsuit, tuck a snugly fitting T-shirt into the tights. Then *really* look at yourself in a full-length mirror.

Concentrate on your bone structure — from under the bust down to your knees. *Don't* immediately classify yourself as curvy because you see lots of soft lines. Is the curviness an actual contour, or is it just excess flesh?

Run your hands firmly against your rib cage and over your hips. Do you go in and out at the waist? Is a lot of your extra weight on your hips and at the tops of your thighs? **You have a curvy body shape.**

When you run your hands firmly against your rib cage and

hips is there only a slight indent for your waist? Look in the mirror; in spite of the extra flesh, do your contours have a straight up and down look about them? **You have a straight body shape.**

CURVY BODY SHAPE
With curvy features and a curvy body, you are totally curvy.
Look back at picture 1. Is this you?

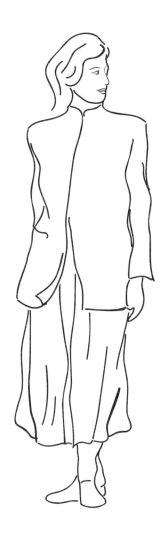

- **You have a round, oval, pear or heart-shaped face.**
- **You have sloping shoulders.**
- **You are softly waisted.**
- **Your hips and thighs have a curvaceous, feminine look.**

Complement curvy shapes with fluid, curvy lines, softer fabrics and swirly patterns.

STRAIGHT BODY SHAPE

With straight features and a straight body, you fall into the totally straight category.

Look back at picture 2. Is this you?

- **You have an oblong, square, diamond or triangular face shape.**
- **Your shoulders are *probably* straight** (don't be side-tracked if they are sloping — if your body and face are straight, simply get those shoulders in line by straightening them with pads!).
- **You have little or no waist.**
- **Your hips and thighs have a straighter, more masculine look than the curvaceous, curvy body shape.**

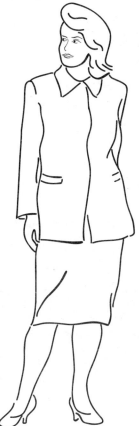

Straight shapes need straighter, crisper lines, firmer fabrics and geometric patterns.

You could also be a combination of shapes.

BIG TIPS
Know your body shape

SOFT/STRAIGHT SHAPE

Someone with curvy features and a straight body has a soft/straight shape (soft on top, straight from the ribcage down).
Look back at picture 3. Is this you?

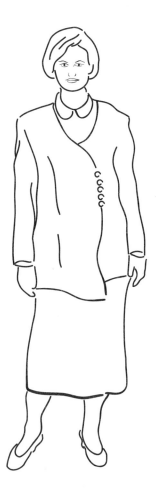

- **You have a round, oval or heart-shaped face.**
- **Your shoulders are *probably* sloping.**
- **You have little or no waist.**
- **Your hips and thighs have a straight, more masculine look than the curvaceous, curvy body shape.**

Necklines and accessories will look best if they have a softened look, and from below the bust, clothes with a straighter line will hang better on your frame.

STRAIGHT/SOFT SHAPE

With straight facial bone structure and a curvy body shape, you fall into the straight/soft category (straight at the top and curvy below).

Look back at picture 4. Is this you?

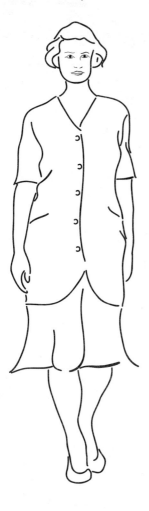

- **You have straight facial features — oblong, square, diamond or triangular.**
- **Your shoulders are *probably* straight.**
- **You are softly waisted.**
- **Your hips and thighs have a curvaceous, feminine look.**
- **You may be straight on top with a curvy, pear-shaped hip (see page 112).**

Necklines and accessories with a crisp, angular, more tailored look will suit you best and, from the rib-cage down, softer, more fluid shapes will hang better on your frame.

I hope you've now identified your basic body shape. Here are one or two common sub-types of those shapes.

CURVY LINE — ARE YOU PEAR-SHAPED?

When you buy separates:

1. Do you buy the same size top as bottom?
2. Do you buy one or more sizes larger for your hips?

If you answered (1) your body is a figure eight and is totally curvy. If you answered (2) your body is pear-shaped. (If your hips take one size bigger, you are a conference pear; if you take two or more sizes bigger, you're a comice!)

Women with this type of figure have a great waistline. If you were ever slim, I'm sure you remember with nostalgia that slim waist. When you put on weight you still have a waist, but the problem is that if you show it off, you just emphasise your bust and hips. So, even though it's tempting to show off such a good feature, *don't do it*. You need to create the illusion of long, vertical lines by adding width to your shoulders and elongating your body.

Try creating a soft, straight line to carry the eye down, elongate yourself and make yourself look taller and slimmer. To be flattering on your curvy hips, particularly if you have good, shapely legs, your skirts need to be tapered.

When you were slimmer, you may have looked good with a blouse tucked in and a belt fastened tight. *I implore you not to attempt this look now.* I frequently see large women tightly belted into a full, dirndl skirt and I'm afraid they look like a sack of potatoes tied in the middle. *You really must avoid this at all costs.* Instead, opt for the flattering tulip skirt, flared skirt or softly-pleated straight skirt.

If you are pear-shaped, you may have to buy skirts and trousers one or two sizes too big in the waist to get them to fit well on the hips. This is far better than going for a garment which is comfortable round the waist, but pulls on the hips. You can always have the waistband taken in, or buy clothes with elasticated waistbands. If you buy a perfectly straight skirt it is easy to have it tapered — it will make the world of difference to the way you look.

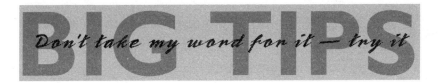

BIG TIPS
Don't take my word for it — try it

Top tips for curves and pears:
- **Avoid tailored jackets.** Wear a camisole over your skirt with a soft jacket, or a blouse worn open as a jacket.
- **Create a streamlined, straighter look, but to complement those curves aim for a softened line.**
- **If you are low-waisted, trousers and skirts will fit better if you have them lifted** — at the front only. Get a tailor to do this for you.

- **Jackets are best worn long,** to draw the eye down, for a leaner look. Make sure your jacket finishes below the widest part of your hips — even more vital for the pear-shaped.

- **Overblouses are invaluable.** A short overblouse gives a waisted, blouson look and is great for a curvy figure. Pear-shapes need longer overblouses, finishing below the widest part of your hips.

- **You need trousers in softly-textured materials such as fine wool or silk jersey — they will flatter but not cling to your curvy hips. Avoid straight-cut, tailored trousers in tightly-woven or heavy fabrics, such as corduroy.** The wider the bottom of the leg, the shorter and fatter you will look — so only wear flowing palazzo pants (preferably with a long waistcoat) if you are tall. If you have slim ankles, harem pants will look great on you. Whatever top you wear should end below where your hips are widest. Trousers work well teamed with long tops (overblouse, tunic, sweater or T-shirt) or with a matching long waistcoat, cardigan or jacket.

- Pear-shaped women often tell me they don't like wearing shoulder pads as they feel big enough without them — in fact, they are an absolute must, to balance your body and make your waist look smaller. **Shoulder pads should bring your shoulders out in line with your hips,** so the bigger your hips, the wider the pads should be. Still not sure? Put a pad on one shoulder only, put on a blouse and look at yourself in a mirror — can you see how much slimmer you look on the side with the pad? The best way to wear shoulder pads is to have Velcro stitched into your clothes and the pads (or use stick-on Velcro). The lazy way is to anchor the narrow part of the pad under your bra strap to keep it in place.

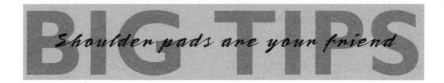

BIG TIPS

Shoulder pads are your friend

- **If you are pear-shaped, see if you can buy a suit as separates,** because you need the skirt one or more sizes bigger than the jacket. Remember this, too: if a jacket's the right size for your bust and long enough to create a straight look, it's probably too small on your hips. You may need to buy the jacket a size larger to be more flattering to your shape — you'll just need bigger shoulder pads to balance the look.
- **If you are pear-shaped and like patterns, keep them to your top half** — it's visually more slimming. Avoid light or shiny fabrics and fussy pocket details below the waist.

The acid test

Have I persuaded you to go out and try to achieve this streamlined, but curvy, look? I guarantee that you will suddenly find, without the scales moving, that you have dropped pounds. Many of my clients have been sceptical at first, but I don't mind — I've seen it and know that it works.

STRAIGHT LINE — ARE YOU HEART-SHAPED?

When you buy separates:

1. Do you buy the same size top as bottom?
2. Do you buy tops one or more sizes larger?

If your answer was (1) your body is totally straight. If your answer was (2) your body is heart-shaped.

A heart-shaped body is easy to recognise: big-busted and thick-waisted, these women frequently have amazingly slim thighs and good legs.

The main feature of a straight body is that it has little or no waist. Blouson styles look good on straight body shapes as they create the illusion of a waist. The blouson effect brings the eye down to the straight hips and thus has an elongating, slimming effect.

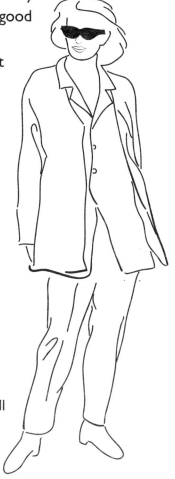

With your long leg line, all trousers will look good on you, from classic, tailored ones to jeans, leggings to flares.

Top tips for straight shapes:

- **If your shoulders are very straight, try wearing thin shoulder pads to fill them out slightly, making them wider than your hips.** Garments will then drape to give the illusion of a waist.
- **Overblouses teamed with straight or straight-pleated skirts are slimming** on a straight figure, as this style hides the absence of waist.
- **If you have slim, shapely legs, make the most of them by wearing a well-fitted, straight skirt, to the knee or just below.** Don't expect to buy a skirt that will fit you perfectly — you'll probably have to buy them at least one or two sizes too big to get the waist big enough for comfort. Then take in the hips to highlight your slim legs.
- **Trousers look much better on large women with straight hips than those with curvy hips.** Elasticated waistbands, to accommodate your thicker waist, are better than going up a size, when the trousers would probably need taking in at the hip. Wear any long-line top over your trousers.

Top tips for heart-shapes:

- **Blouses look best not tucked in.** A blouse over a straight skirt is one of your best looks. To be most flattering, a blouse should be slightly tapered under the bust and fit snugly over the hips.
- **Shorter skirts, reaching just below the knee, look good on this figure, particularly when teamed with a longer jacket.**
- The eye acts like a barcode scanner and stops at a

horizontal line, so **don't wear sleeves that stop at your bust line,** as this will draw attention to it and make it appear bigger. **Also be careful about pockets or details on blouses at the bust line.**

● Most heart-shaped women have broad shoulders and rarely need shoulder pads, but **if your shoulders are sloped you may need just a little padding to lift them.**

● **If you have a very big bust, a handbag rather than a shoulder bag will look more streamlined.**

● **Single-breasted rather than double-breasted jackets will minimise the bust.**

● **If you like patterns, keep them to your bottom half.**

● **Dolman sleeves flatter a large bust.**

Swimwear

Choosing swimwear is tricky for most large women because it's so difficult to hide any problem areas — swimsuits leave little to the imagination. Start by choosing the right size — usually one size smaller than your dress size since, if you swim a lot and it's not a close fit, it's likely to become baggy and need replacing. If it bulges, cuts in or rides up, it's too small.

There are some general hints on what to look for:

● **One-piece suits** or, for tall sizes 16-20, a two-piece with a waist-high bikini bottom

● **Deep colours and minimal patterns**

● **Matt, not shiny, fabric**

● **Medium-cut leg**

- **Vertical stripes and panels minimise the stomach, as do blouson styles and diagonal stripes**
- **Built-in stomach control panels**

For specific figure types:

Pear-shaped Choose styles that draw the eye away from the hips, with colour and pattern on top and plain colour around the hips. If you have a small bust, look for swimsuits with detail at the bustline — bandeau tops, ruffles or gathers. Avoid skirted swimsuits.

Heart-shaped Make sure the swimsuit has good bust support: choose an underwired bra top and substantial straps. A good tip to minimise your upper half is to choose swimsuits which have little or no detail at the bust with pattern at the waist or below, if at all.

Moving On

These are just some of the things I've found useful in helping my clients arrive at the best look for their shape. Now it's time for you to try some of the ideas out for yourself — I hope you have fun. Oh, and another tip — keep your eyes open and look at how other people with your body shape dress. If they look good, adopt the look for yourself. If they don't, the knowledge you now have should give you some clues as to why, and you can avoid making the same mistake.

I think knowing the style to suit your body shape is the most important thing, but colour can also do a lot for your image and the visual impact you create. Next, we're going to take a look at what colours can do for you and which ones you, personally, should look out for.

CHAPTER SIX

Living with Colour

HOW TO WEAR *ALL* COLOURS SUCCESSFULLY

E ver been colour analysed? Do you long to be? Scared that it might mean getting rid of all the clothes in your wardrobe? Or do you simply wonder what it's all about? It's not easy to explain everything in a book — I really need to have you in front of my mirror, trying colours up against your face, but I'm going to do my best to explain how it works and show you how to find out which colours work best for you.

A Background in Colour

Image consultants like myself train initially as colour analysts, and most (other than corporate image consultants) spend a large proportion of their time doing colour analysis. So you might well expect image consultants to say that colour is more important than style. I believe, however, that if you wear a garment which is a superb colour for you but the style is wrong, it will not flatter you at all. And the larger you are, the less flattering it will be.

In my opinion, matching your clothes to your *shape* is the most important consideration. If you wear a good style you can make it work for you, even if the colour is not one of your best — a scarf in a good colour, some jewellery or even the clever use of make-up can make all the difference. After all, think of the LBD (Little Black Dress) or black suit. Although many people wear black, how many would honestly say it is perfect for them? Often they will look stunning, not *because* of their black outfit, but in spite of it, through the imaginative use of accessories. More on those later.

Colour Analysis — How it Works

A colour analyst is a specialist in her field (most colour analysts are women). She aims to diagnose your colour strengths and weaknesses. To do this she looks at your skin colour, the colour of your eyes and, where possible, the natural colour of your hair. Then, by draping your shoulders with coloured scarves, she demonstrates the effects of 'right' and 'wrong' colours on your appearance. Your 'best' colours are the colours that look really good by your face — these would be for blouses, dresses, T-shirts, collars, scarves, necklaces, earrings and so on. Don't worry if at first you don't see what she means — when you're in front of that mirror, being draped with all kinds of colours, it gradually becomes as clear as day that a certain 'family' of colours is better for you than another. I call this 'family' your *colour direction*.

Right and wrong

The wrong colours heighten any imperfections. Your skin may look ruddy or sallow, lines and shadows may appear — which age you — and any facial features you are not happy about come leaping out at you. Strong shades of the wrong colours stand out more than your face, which means people notice your clothes *before* they see you.

A good colour next to your face will facilitate that all-important eye contact and get you the attention and respect you need to put across whatever you are trying to communicate. In the 'right' colours you can immediately see how they clarify and smooth your skin, minimise shadows and lines and give you a healthy glow. The people you meet notice *you* first, make eye contact and start relating to you, *then* notice what you are wearing.

Some of you may be reluctant to be colour analysed because you think it will restrict your choice of colour. Are you worried that you'll be told never to wear navy again, when you have a wardrobe full of navy clothes? Dread being told to go on a colour diet of mustard yellow and shocking pink? Have no fear, there are blues, greens, reds, pinks and even navies for everyone.

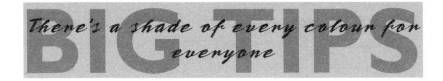

BIG TIPS
There's a shade of every colour for everyone

It is the depth, tone and clarity — the shades — of the colours, and where on your body you wear them, that is important. If your instinct tells you that the colours of your clothes don't always work for you, or that your wardrobe is a complete jumble of colours, why not have a go at colour analysis?

About analysis

A full analysis with a qualified analyst takes anything from one to two and a half hours. Each analyst or company has a different approach, but most use anything from 80 to 150 different coloured scarves as drapes. Your analyst will show you which tones suit you best and give you a shopping wallet of appropriate colour samples (somewhere between 30 and 48). She'll show you how to use your samples when you're shopping to find the colours which are best by your face; which are best for a jacket or accessories; how to mix and match your colours; and how to create a versatile wardrobe full of co-ordinating clothes.

Many men also seek the advice of a colour analyst or image consultant. They usually want to establish the best colours for shirts and ties in relation to their suits; whether to go for single- or double-breasted jackets; what glasses would suit them best; how to style their hair, and so on (turn to Chapter Nine for some ideas on this).

You're probably right

I have been an image consultant for ten years and I have seen hundreds of men and women. Rest assured — very few sessions involve a complete rethink of a client's wardrobe. Many women, and men too, have a good natural sense of which colours suit them and have been buying their clothes accordingly for years. Although some sessions pinpoint where clients have been going wrong, it's quite common for the analyst to confirm where they have been going right! But even if you have been getting it right, it's fascinating to try to understand *why*, and an analysis will help you to add interesting colours to your wardrobe — ones you've never thought of wearing before.

The Seasonal Approach

When colour analysis was first introduced into this country in the early 1980s, seasonal analysis was the exclusive method used. I'll explain what it's all about later, but first let me tell you a bit about the background to it.

Colour analysis is not a new invention. In Germany in the late 1930s, Johannes Itten, a master of the Bauhaus School of Art, noted that when he sent a class of students out to paint, they would always make the same choice of colour palettes. Itten began to study these habits and noticed that his students seemed to choose colours which were in harmony with their individual colouring, and they frequently dressed accordingly too.

He found that the students who had 'cool' colouring painted using mainly 'cool' tones. Students who had 'warm' colouring painted using 'warm' tones. Those who had a bright look about their skin, eyes and hair used vibrant colours; others who had a softer, muted look about them tended to paint with dusty, hazy colours.

The Bauhaus School of Art fled Germany with the rise of Hitler and settled on the West Coast of America. Some while later, the papers that Itten had written on this subject led to further investigation and the development of the first method of colour analysis, whereby people were categorised as having warm, cool, bright or muted colouring.

The seasons

You will very often find that the clothes you rarely wear or feel unsure about turn out to be in colours which are not among your best. The reason you so frequently get colours *right* is because *colour is subjective*. As Itten found with his art students, you will be drawn to colours that complement your hair and skin. The first colour analysts took the warm, cool, bright and muted categories and labelled them Winter, Summer, Autumn and Spring. The first colour analysts divided people into these categories and some companies still do so, although variations have developed.

If you are told you are a Winter, Summer, Autumn or Spring person, it has nothing to do with when you were born, but is because you look best in colours that nature provides at that time of the year.

In spring, you see bright splashes of colours. The grass has a particularly vivid shade of green, the flowers — crocuses, daffodils, irises — are bright, delicate shades. Anyone who looks good in warm, light, bright shades of colour is described as 'Spring'.

In summer, colours tend to have a softer look. Think of the soft shadings of sweet peas or pansies with their gradations of colour, the colours of a summer sunset — the myriad shadings of pink, blue and delicate, hazy, blue-greys. People who come to life in these cool, soft, muted tones are called 'Summer'.

Next, imagine walking through a wood on a fine autumn morning. Think of the glowing colours of all those crunchy autumn leaves, the chestnut shades, the lovely russet tones, the rich, warm greens and browns that surround you. These warm, intense shades look good on people who are described as 'Autumn'.

You can wear all colours successfully, if you know how

Now picture yourself standing on top of a hill in the middle of winter. Visualise a lone tree, starkly outlined in the distance, its black silhouette standing out in strong contrast to the snow-covered ground. Imagine a pine tree, its dark, blue-green leaves against a clear sky, and a holly bush nearby with vivid, emerald green leaves and bright, scarlet berries. These all have bold, high-contrast colours — perfect for the 'Winter' person.

Mixing your metaphors

Although it certainly works, I find the strictly seasonal approach to colour too rigid. It can also become extremely boring. For example, Springs and Autumns are told *never* to wear black or white; Winters should *never* wear brown or cream; Summers should *never* wear bright colours, and so on. Colour should be exciting. You want to know *how* to wear the colours you like and the colours that are in the shops — not simply to be told not to wear them. The restrictions of the purely seasonal approach are even more frustrating if you have a problem finding clothes you like, which flatter your shape — and which *fit.*

Most colour analysts today take a more flexible approach. They introduce their clients to their best colours and then show them how to wear *all* colours — in other words, they tell you the rules and then teach you how to bend them to suit yourself.

BIG TIPS

If it goes with other things you have — buy it

Knowing your best colour direction is useful. It helps you plan a wardrobe you can mix and match. But I prefer to follow a simple rule of thumb: it must go with at least two, preferably three, other things in your existing wardrobe. Otherwise, DO NOT BUY IT. When I tell this to a new client I am frequently asked 'But where do I start? Does this mean I'll never be able to buy anything new as it won't match what I've already got?' In fact, it's very easy to do. You start with the items in your wardrobe which you know look great on you and buy things to team with these. If you see a blouse you like, buy it only if it will go with a couple of skirts you already own. Before you buy a new suit, be sure that the skirt will go with blouses you already own and the jacket will tone with other skirts of yours. Gradually the selection in your wardrobe expands — it's an exciting challenge, and it works!

Some colour companies never use the seasonal terminology, only the descriptive terms — warm/cool; bright/muted; dark/light. Others, including me, combine the seasonal and descriptive approach. I feel it gives the best of both worlds.

Getting Down to Business

The most important point to establish in colour analysis is whether you are a 'cool' person or a 'warm' person. The only way to ensure a well co-ordinated wardrobe is to have either predominantly cool or warm colours; not both.

Next, you need to establish your colour direction — that's 'bright' or 'muted', 'light' or 'deep' — and which is your season. This is where a book has its limitations! Even if you have an idea of your category, reading a book can never replace an analysis. The only way really to assess the best colours for you is to see your local colour analyst. But in the meantime, read on, and enjoy trying to work it out for yourself.

Find Your Colour Direction

The questions below are designed to help you find your colour direction. Don't think for too long about any of them; answer quickly and spontaneously and you should get an accurate result.

Warm or cool?

If you are not sure which colours are warm and which are cool you are not alone — the box below should help to clarify this.

	Warm colours (golden based)	Cool colours (blue based)
Red	orangey reds e.g. flame	blue reds e.g. cherry
Green	yellowy greens e.g. leaf green	blue greens e.g. emerald
Blue	greeny blues e.g. teal	rich blues e.g. royal blue
Pink	peachy tones e.g. coral pink	blue pinks e.g. fuchsia

1. Open your make-up case or drawer. Which of the following groups do most of your lipsticks fall into?
   a) Pinky tones; fuchsias; blue-reds; red burgundies.
   b) Peachy-coppery tones; soft brown; orange reds; brown burgundies.
2. Which of the these neutral shades do you prefer yourself in?
   a) White or soft white.
   b) Ivory or cream.
3. In the sun, wearing a low-factor lotion do you:
   a) burn easily?
   b) tan gradually?
4. Do you prefer yourself in:
   a) black?
   b) brown?
5. Do you prefer yourself in:
   a) royal blue?
   b) teal blue?
6. Open your wardrobe. Which colours predominate?
   a) Fuchsias; magentas; emeralds; blue reds; primary colours.
   b) Golden peachy tones; warm orange reds; yellowy greens.

Is your colour direction warm or cool?

Rating:
If you scored 4 or more (a)s you look best in cool tones.
If you scored 4 or more (b)s you look best in warm tones.

Soft/muted or bright/vibrant?
Some people can make an immediate decision on this next question. If you can, fine, if not, don't worry about it.

1. Look in your wardrobe. Which of the following best describes your clothes?

   a) Most are brightly coloured.

   b) There is a soft quality to their colouring.

2. When you wear more than one colour, which do you prefer?

   a) High contrast, such as navy with red or orange.

   b) A more blended, quieter look.

Is your colour direction bright or muted?

Rating:

If you answered (a) to both, you look best in vibrant colours and your colour direction is bright.

If you answered (b) to both, you look best in soft tones and your colour direction is muted.

Deep or light?

When you choose tops — blouses, sweaters, T-shirts — do you prefer:

   a) mainly dark shades?

   b) mainly light colours?

Is your colour direction deep or light?

Rating:

If you answered (a) your colour direction is deep.

If you answered (b) your colour direction is light.

Now you should know whether you are bright or soft, deep or light, cool or warm. Whatever your other answers, if you think you are 'cool' you will either be Winter or Summer; if you think you are 'warm', you are either Spring or Autumn. The following quiz should confirm that you are on the right track.

The warm/cool quiz

Again, don't think about this too long, and if you fit into more than one category, don't worry.

Imagine yourself wearing a navy jacket. Tick which groups of colours you would choose for a blouse or top to make your face come to life (tick as many as you think apply):

a) Bright, high-contrast colours — white; clear, bright red; emerald green; bright fuchsia; bright magenta.

b) Bright but lighter tones — ivory; orangey red; lime green; peach; bright, tealy blue.

c) Truly warm colours — orange; orangey red; bright gold; coral.

d) Intensely cool, blue toned-colours, but not as bright as (a) — fuchsia; blue reds; blue greens.

e) Light, soft, pastel shades — candy floss pink; baby blue; pale blue-green.

f) Light, warm colours — light, peachy tones; light, yellowy green; light aqua.

g) Muted, softened tones, with a 'dusted' quality about them — a soft medley of pinks, blues, greens.

h) Soft, monochromatic colours — blends of beige, browns and rusts; soft golds and mustards; soft peachy tones; camel; creams.

i) Deep, warm, intense colours — rusts; deep orange; dark, olive green; strong, deep teal.

j) Deep, cool, bold colours — burgundy; pine green; royal blue; deep magenta.

Rating:

If you ticked some of the following, you are warm: b, c, f, h, i (Autumn/Spring).

If you ticked some of the following, you are cool: a, d, e, g, j (Winter/Summer).

I'm sure by now you will have decided whether you are 'cool' or 'warm'. I hope you have also managed to decide whether your colour direction is 'bright' or 'muted', 'light' or 'deep'. Now on to some of the finer points on colour.

The controversy over black

Many large women wear black because they think it's flattering and makes them look slimmer. This is true — a dark colour makes an object recede and so it's great to wear as a skirt or trousers. Pale colours reflect the light and are more noticeable, that's why your rear looks bigger in white or pale trousers.

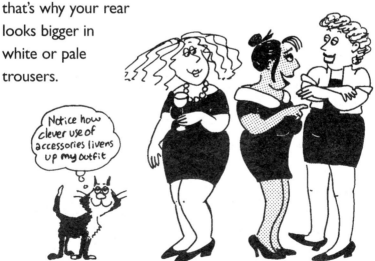

Notice how clever use of accessories livens up my outfit

Black trousers and skirts are fine for everyone, but black by your face is another matter. It looks best on people with deep colouring. And, even with the right colouring, handle black with care once you are over forty. If you don't have deep colouring, black by your face can make you look pale, tired and drained, and people's attention is drawn to the depth of colour rather than to you. However, as I said before, you can wear black and other dark colours successfully provided you wear one of your best colours against your face, perhaps in a scarf, collar or jewellery.

BIG TIPS

Make black work for you

The lower the neckline on an LBD, the easier it is to make it look good as the black is further from your face.

Here are a few ideas on how to wear that LBD:

- **If you are bright** — wear bright colours by your face, such as bright, clear red, blue or green.
- **If you are muted** — wear softened, hazy tones by your face to soften the effect, such as warm blends of peaches, rusts and creams, or soft, cool blends of blues, smoky greys, pinks and greens.
- **If you are warm** — wear golden tones by your face to warm up the black, such as orange, mustard, lime green or teal.
- **If you are cool** — wear cool tones by your face, such as magenta, cerise, emerald green or cherry red.

- **If you are light** — wear light tones by your face, such as cool, powdery blues, greens and pinks, or warm, light tones of peach and ivory.
- **If you are deep** and under forty — black probably looks wonderful on you. Over forty? Look objectively at yourself — you may need to soften the black with a deep, rich colour, perhaps burgundy, royal blue or deep magenta.

White versus cream

White or soft white will clarify a 'cool' skin and make it look vibrant and alive, while cream or ivory will deaden it and may make you look sallow. If you have a 'warm' skin, cream or ivory will enhance your skin tone and be more flattering than white, which will always look slightly clinical on you.

Gold versus silver

I have lots more to say on this subject in the next chapter. For now, remember that if you are a 'cool' person, silver will look better against your skin tone than gold. If you are 'warm', then gold will look better than silver.

Bending the Rules

Each season, certain colours are more fashionable than others. If, like most women, you like to look up-to-date, let me show you how to wear all colours successfully.

Frequently, you will find clothes in styles that suit you, but which are not available in any of your best colours. Provided you actually like the colour, once you know your colour direction there is always a way to wear it. Look back at how

I have suggested wearing black and do the same for any shade which is not one of your best.

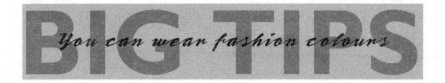

BIG TIPS
You can wear fashion colours

For example, say the current season's high fashion colours are mainly muted and warm, perhaps khakis, beiges or olives. That's wonderful for anyone who looks their best in muted/warm shades, but not for people who are at their best in deep colours. The solution is to wear a blouse or sweater in a deep colour by your face and keep the muted/warm shades away from your face — perhaps as a jacket or a waistcoat. If you've found a fabulous dress in a muted, warm shade — it's the perfect style and the price is right — wear a deep-coloured scarf to blend and contrast with it, or perhaps jet beads or other jewellery so that you have a deep colour by your face to give you that all-important eye-contact. If you look your best in bright colours, wear a bright blouse, sweater or jewellery. Just imagine the impact of a red blouse with a khaki jacket or, if you are 'cool', a magenta blouse with an olive jacket.

Make-up Colours

As with clothes, your make-up colours can enhance or detract from your look. When you read Chapter Three and did project three did you notice that most of the make-up you rarely use falls into one category — either 'warm' or 'cool' shades? As with clothes, once you have established whether you are 'warm' or 'cool', all you need is either 'warm' or 'cool' make-up.

Here are a few guidelines:

Cool

All your make-up should have a blue base: avoid yellow/beige/golden undertones.

- **Lipstick** Fuchsia and all shades of pink which are not peachy; red; burgundies; blue, or true, reds which don't turn orange.
- **Eyeshadows** Greys — from silver grey through to charcoal; blues — from navy through to cornflower; greens — any blue-green such as emerald or jade; purples and violets.
- **Blusher** All shades of pink which have no brown in them.
- **Foundation** Pinky, rosy tones; nothing beige-based.

Warm

All your make-up should have a golden base: no blue undertone.

- **Lipstick** Coppery shades, such as bronze and russet; brown burgundies; all pinks which have no blue tone to them; all orange shades and orange reds; peachy shades.
- **Eyeshadows** All the autumnal shades — leafy, yellowy greens; olive greens; yellows and golds; russets; browns of any description; teal blues, aqua blues, purples and violets.
- **Blusher** All shades of browny, fudge-coloured pinks; corally pinks.
- **Foundation** Beige based tones; nothing pink-based.

I'm sure you can now see the relevance of knowing whether you are 'warm' or 'cool' and what your general colour direction is. I hope the world of colour has opened up for you and you will try some adventurous things when you next go shopping. I'm going to move on to accessories now — because all the details count.

CHAPTER SEVEN

All the Etceteras

EVERY DETAIL TELLS A STORY

I'm sure I've drummed in enough by now how important your appearance is in making a good impression and grabbing that first eye-contact. You'll soon see that if you can make eye-contact, you'll get better reactions from everyone you speak to — employers, employees, partner, child, parent, bank manager — even a salesperson when you take something back to a store for a refund! As I've already pointed out, eye-contact isn't simply a question of looking directly at somebody, although this is important. Your whole appearance, and especially your shoulders, face and head, must be visually appealing. One of the best ways to catch people's eye (and retain it) is by using accessories.

The Importance of Accessories

This story, which happened to a client of mine, Joy, shows what you can achieve with accessories.

Joy is personal assistant to Mr. Hawkins, director of a large shipping company. One day last summer he rang to tell her that he was caught in traffic on the M25 and would be at least half an hour late for an important meeting. He told her that as she knew nearly as much about the business in hand as he did, he would like her to apologise on his behalf and start the meeting for him — a flattering suggestion, showing how much he appreciated her abilities.

Joy is in her early thirties although she looks much younger. She is 5ft 1in and a size 18. As it was a hot day, she had come to work in just a skirt, sleeveless blouse and sandals, wearing no make-up — and how she regretted it now! In her own words, she looked barely capable of setting out the notes in the boardroom and putting the kettle on for tea.

Luckily, she knew enough about the importance of first impressions to scout around her colleagues for more suitable clothes. She borrowed a navy jacket which just about fitted, but at least covered her bare arms, and found a pair of earrings in her handbag. Another colleague lent her a brooch for the jacket. She always kept make-up in her desk drawer so quickly put on some eyeliner, mascara and lipstick. She glanced at herself in the mirror. A definite improvement, totally marred by her feet. They looked ready for a day on the beach, not a business meeting. She swapped shoes with a colleague and with her wide, size 4D feet crammed into a pair of narrow, size 5B court shoes she grimly got on with the job in hand.

As everyone was entering the boardroom, Joy heard one of the managers remark, 'It's good to have someone not only capable of running things, but who looks so capable and efficient too.' Joy smiled to herself and knew that the effort had been worthwhile.

Joy used to think that it didn't matter how she dressed if she wasn't seeing clients. Now she realises the importance of going to work looking the part every day, whatever the weather. She is also aware of the impact a jacket, a little make-up and accessories can have, giving her that extra air of authority.

Emergency Makeover Kit

My advice is that for the one day when, perhaps, you didn't bother, you ensure that you keep in your office:

- **Make-up** — lipstick, eyeliner and mascara at the very least. Perhaps also concealer, blusher and powder
- **A classic pair of shoes** in a dark, neutral colour
- **A jacket** — again in a neutral colour. Wearing a jacket always adds a professional look to a skirt or dress. Surveys show that a dark colour carries far more authority than a light colour
- **A few accessories** — whatever appeals to you most: a brooch, earrings, perhaps a scarf
- **Shoe polish**
- **Clothes brush**

Chic Short-cut

Have you been to Rome? Paris? Geneva? What strikes me about all Continental women is the way they accessorise. The quality of their accessories is always outstanding and makes the clothes they wear look a million dollars even if they were bought at a local chainstore.

If a Parisian woman needs to look good and can't afford a new outfit, she'll buy a new blouse, polish up an old but expensive pair of shoes and matching handbag, and accessorise an old outfit with a piece of exquisite jewellery. She would *never* be seen in scuffed shoes or without tights. Her hair is always in place and her make-up discreet and immaculate.

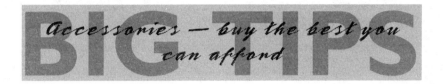

BIG TIPS

Accessories — buy the best you can afford

Getting accessories right can be tricky. Too many accessories give a frivolous impression but, in fact, most women under-accessorise — probably afraid of looking OTT. OK, we all know that one elegant woman who rarely wears accessories or make-up, yet always looks poised. But for most of us poor mortals, wearing too few accessories (apart from when in sports gear), actually makes us look understated — a sign of lack of confidence and low self-esteem.

Of course, there will always be a season when the fashion pundits decide that accessories will be minimal but, other than this, there are some generally accepted principles on how to accessorise successfully. To find out where you stand in the accessories stakes, try this quiz.

The Accessories Quiz

Give yourself one point for each of the following:
- **Wearing make-up**

- **Wearing glasses** (even though you may have to wear them, they are such a big focal point that they do count as an accessory)
- **Each piece of jewellery you have on,** such as a watch, a brooch, a necklace, a hair accessory: one point only for a pair of earrings, two rings worn on one finger and so on.
- **A jacket**
- **Contrasting buttons**
- **Wearing more than one colour,** for example:

  A suit with matching blouse counts as one point only (for the jacket)

  A suit with a contrasting blouse counts as two points — one for the jacket plus another for the blouse

  A suit with a multi-coloured, contrasting blouse would count as one point for the jacket plus two points for the blouse

  A suit with brass buttons would warrant an extra point for the buttons

  An unmatched suit would warrant an extra point for a contrasting skirt
- **Scarf or neck detail** (bow or frill on blouse)
- **Belt**
- **Patterned or coloured tights**
- **Detail on shoes** (sling back, peep toe, bow etc.)
- **Clear nail polish** (two points for bright red or anything extreme about the nails)

Look in the mirror now and count up the points.

Results:

If you are 5ft 1in or under you should be aiming for nine to ten points.

5ft 2in–5ft 6in: aim for ten to twelve points.

5ft 7in or over: aim for eleven to thirteen points.

Under eight points? You are definitely under-dressed. Add something. A piece of jewellery, a scarf or perhaps a handkerchief in a jacket pocket.

Fourteen points or more? *Subtract something!*

Obviously, this is only general guidance. You may be 5ft1in or less *and* have a big, bouncy personality, in which case, on the accessories scale, ten points — and even eleven — would look great. More, or larger, accessories, or bright nail varnish which would look garish on a quieter individual, will look really good on you.

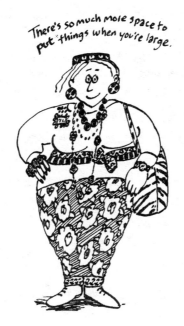

There's so much more space to put things when you're large.

The Art of Accessorising

Your accessories need to relate either to something else you are wearing or to each other. In other words, if you have silver buttons on your blazer, then wear silver earrings, not gold. Or if you want to wear gold earrings, wear a brooch with both silver and gold in it to tie them all together. If you are wearing a green blouse, you could match the colour with a green handkerchief in your jacket pocket, or perhaps with green earrings.

Jewellery

Believe it or not, I've actually heard of women changing all the buttons on their clothes to match their jewellery because they have been told that they are 'warm' and look best in gold or that they are 'cool' and look best in silver. While that's a good rule of thumb, sticking to only one metal for jewellery is far too rigid (and boring — not to mention the hassle of changing buttons!).

Mary, one of my clients, is a part-time secretary in her early forties. She was told that as she was 'warm' and therefore a 'gold person', not only should she change the buttons on all her suits and blouses but also *never* wear shoes, handbags or belts with silver trimmings. She was even advised to dispense with her new briefcase because it had a silver clasp. What nonsense! No one needs to go to such extremes.

Fortunately, the frames of her glasses were gold and I advised her to make sure that any jewellery she wore near her face had some gold content. I also suggested that she look for earrings, brooches and necklaces in mixed metals. This way, whatever the colour of buttons or metal trimmings on her clothes, bags and shoes, they would still blend in with her other accessories.

Top tips

- **Pearls** are wonderful. Some have a lovely creamy, ivory tone, others are nearly white or have a pink sheen. You should know by now whether you are cool or warm and whether your white is soft white/white (cool) or cream/ivory (warm). Don't get too pedantic about it, but if you can find pearls which have the best tone for you, buy them, you'll look fabulous.

- **Rings and bracelets** draw attention to your hands. Great, if you have attractive, well-groomed hands. If you have podgy fingers, avoid chunky rings — they'll emphasise them. If you put weight on, have rings re-sized — too-tight rings don't look or feel good.

- **Bracelets** — and watches — should be loose enough to slide around easily. Be careful with chunky, cuff-style bracelets, which can make arms look shorter and dumpy; on the other hand, thin, delicate chains may be lost on a thick wrist.

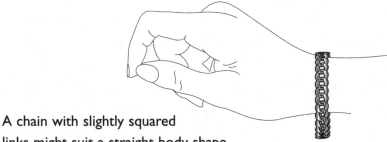

A chain with slightly squared
links might suit a straight body shape.

- **A brooch** finishes off an outfit. But if you have a large bust, beware of wearing too much jewellery on top: choose a brooch or necklace, not both. Don't wear a brooch too low on your lapel, it will draw attention to your chest. Wear it higher to draw the eye up to your face.

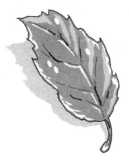

This brooch would suit all face shapes. It is a wonderful blend of straight lines and curves.

See also Chapter Four for advice on choosing earrings and necklaces.

Scarves

A scarf can transform an outfit but a lot of large women, particularly those with big busts and/or short necks and double chins, don't like wearing scarves and are right to avoid them like the plague.

However, if you are small-busted and like wearing scarves, they can complement a new outfit or update an old one.

The most useful scarf for all figure types is a long, fairly narrow one to wear inside a coat or jacket for added warmth and colour. If the scarf is long enough, try wearing it tied like a man's tie, only loosely, to keep it in place.

Handbags

Many women have a vast collection of shoes and handbags and are forever adding to it. As fashions come and go, handbag sizes fluctuate. But if you are a large woman — even a short, large woman — a small handbag is always going to look ridiculous. Remember the tips about matching curves with curves and straight lines with straight lines and apply the same theory to handbags. If you have curvy hips, try curvy bags such as drawstrings, or floppy styles. If you have straight hips, go for angular bags, such as a briefcase shape or Kelly bag. If you are curvy and pear-shaped, but decided a straight line suited you in Chapter Five, you'll do best with a bag that's a mix of straight and curvy, or even a totally straight one.

It's quite likely you've homed in on the right shape anyway, in the past, without knowing why. Well, now you know.

Briefcase versus handbag

I see lots of business women carrying both a briefcase and a handbag, and it can look clumsy. Imagine going somewhere for the first time and having to negotiate a door, shake hands, manage your briefcase, hold on to your handbag — and still make a good impression. On the other hand, nothing is worse than needing to go to the toilet at a business meeting and having to take your entire briefcase with you — particularly if you carry half your office around with you.

Rather than use a handbag *and* a briefcase here are three good alternatives:

1. A briefcase-style handbag in which you can keep everything.
2. A woman's briefcase which has a separate, matching clutch bag for your personal items.
3. A conventional briefcase with your personal items in an envelope or clutch bag (the same colour as the briefcase) in one of the compartments of the briefcase.

Negotiating the door and the toilet without clattering or dropping things (even without a briefcase) can be a challenge when you are a large woman; if you use one of the options above, you can slip the small bag out of your briefcase when you go to the toilet and have all you need to hand in a practical purse.

Belts

On most large women, a belt merely highlights an area which is best forgotten. If you have a good waistline, however, try wearing a low-slung belt tied loosely. If it manages not to accentuate your bust and hips, go for it.

Shoes and boots

To me it is self-evident that your shoes, and particularly your heels, are as well taken care of as the rest of your clothes. (I can see you tucking your feet out of sight under the chair as you read this.)

Just because you are large, you don't necessarily have thick ankles or fat legs. Lots of my large clients have slim ankles and very shapely calves. If you are one of these lucky ladies, make the

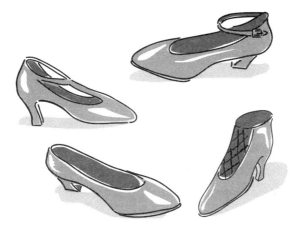

Highlight a well-turned calf with unusual and interesting shoe styles.

most of them. I'm sure you've already twigged that trimmings on shoes, ankle straps, or peep toes revealing brightly varnished nails will all draw attention to your legs and ankles.

If you *do* have thick ankles and calves, obviously *don't* draw attention to your feet by wearing any of the above. Stick to classic, fairly unobtrusive styles such as court shoes.

BIG TIPS
Good legs? Flaunt them

For slim ankles and calves, ankle-length boots are a great idea — team with a calf-length skirt for maximum effect. Just make sure the skirt finishes above or below the point where your calves are widest.

With good legs, you can also invest in long, sexy boots. Worn with a short skirt, or a long one with an alluring slit up the side, this can be a super look (provided those superb legs are not marred by podgy, dimpled knees). Sit in front of a mirror and take a critical look at your knees (or whatever part of your legs is showing) before you decide whether or not the style is for you.

Although flatties are comfortable, a heel, however small, gives you that little bit of extra authority, which is nice to have. The larger you are, the stouter the heel needs to be, otherwise you'll look off-balance.

More and more shops are aware that large women frequently need a wider-fitting shoe, and each season there is a better range. *Never* attempt to buy shoes that aren't wide enough. If your feet hurt, *it shows* in the pained grimace on your face.

Do you drive? In your decent shoes? I'm sure the expression 'down at heel' was in our vocabulary long before cars were invented, but one of the quickest ways of looking 'down at heel' is to drive in good shoes. It doesn't take more than a few minutes to change into driving shoes — keep some in the car specifically. However, *don't forget to change back* before you get out of the car.

My girlfriend, Bobby, was hot-footing it down a crowded St. John's High Road, late for an important interview. Suddenly, she realised she was limping. Looking down, she saw to her horror that one foot was encased in a neat, small-heeled brown court shoe to match her business-like briefcase, while the other (her driving foot) had on a shabby, navy suede, flat slingback. There was obviously an identical odd pair back in the car! She whirled in an about-turn, laddered her tights (but luckily had a spare pair), zoomed back to the car and just made the interview with seconds to spare. She won't do *that* again.

Shoes and colour
Clients often ask me what colour shoes to wear in relation to their outfit. My feeling is that you will always have a well-balanced look if your shoes are the same colour as your hemline, or darker. A dark skirt with white shoes doesn't do anyone any favours.

Hosiery
Nearly every woman, whatever her shape or size, tries to make herself look taller and slimmer (unless she is 5ft 9in plus). To achieve this, your tights or stockings should be the same colour as your hemline, or at least have the same density of colour (it can be lighter — never darker — but it's not as elongating).

BIG TIPS

Keep shoes, legs and hem the same colour

Interestingly, on the catwalk recently, neutral tights were shown with dark shoes and a dark hemline. The media commented on it extensively, but not many women followed the trend; probably because they naturally preferred the lengthening effect of shoes, tights and hemline in one colour.

In my opinion, white or stone shoes really look good only with a white or stone hemline and neutral hosiery. It tends to look tacky if you wear white shoes with dark stockings.

Tights tip

Keep a neutral (skin tone) pair of tights in your office drawer and another pair in your briefcase. They may not always be the perfect choice, but they will go with anything in an emergency.

Tights controversy?

As recently as four or five years ago it was unthinkable for a businesswoman to go without tights, even on the hottest summer day — or for a woman to attend a formal function with 'naked' legs. Now, even at Ascot, hosiery doesn't appear to be essential. But I reckon it's still advisable to wear some if you want to be taken seriously; and, let's face it, however good your legs are, when you're dressed up to the nines, they do look a bit unfinished without tights or stockings.

See also Chapter Three, Foundations Matter.

Coats

Coats aren't strictly accessories, but I want to pass on some general guidelines about choosing them. Remember that, especially in winter, your coat may be the first thing that people notice, so don't ruin a smart outfit by covering it with some old, worn overcoat that you keep bundled up in the back of the car.

Tips on coats

- **Single-breasted styles are more slimming.**
- **Go for long, flowing styles;** and avoid bulky padded jackets.
- If you don't like the restriction of a smart coat, **try a large woollen wrap** instead.
- If you have a belted mac or coat, **tie the belt** at the back, not around the waist. Or, better still, remove the belt and take off the loops.

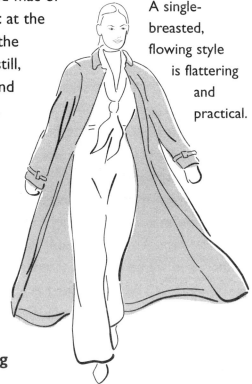

A single-breasted, flowing style is flattering and practical.

- **Dark coloured coats are versatile and slimming —** brighten them up with a brooch or coloured scarf/shawl.
- See advice on page 77 (Chapter Three) for **getting the right fit.**

Weddings and 'Dos'

I am often asked how to accessorise for a wedding. Many people seem to forget their natural instincts and taste and feel they *must* wear hat, bag and shoes in the same colour. There's nothing wrong with this, it can look good, but it isn't strictly necessary. For instance, if your outfit is green and you fancy navy accessories, you could wear them all navy, but what about wearing a green hat that complements the outfit, with just navy shoes and bag? The general rule is to make sure that at least two things (clothes or accessories) are the same colour.

Wedding tips

Look back at Chapter Four for hints on how to buy and wear a hat for that special occasion. And what about budgeting? Think before you buy a dress for a special occasion. How much wear will you get out of it? It may be much better to hire. This applies to a hat for Ascot, too, if you are never likely to wear it again.

Bridal wear

A bride-to-be told me recently that when she went gown hunting with her slim sister, the assistants in one shop assumed that her sister was the one getting married. They seemed surprised that anybody would marry someone her size. How irritating and outrageously rude!

Many specialist bridal shops will make a dress up in a larger size but they rarely have anything bigger than a size 18 for the prospective bride to try on. Looking at magazines doesn't help much either. If you see a gorgeous dress with layers and layers of petticoats on a size 10, 5ft 9in model, do bear in mind that once this is made up into a large size it could make you look like a blancmange.

If you are going to have a gown made but there's nothing to try on in your size, you can get a surprisingly good idea of how a style will look on you by putting just your arms into a dress several sizes too small and letting the material drape in front of you.

Big bridesmaids

If your maids of honour are large, rather than putting them in bridesmaids' dresses choose matching evening dresses (they can wear these for another occasion too — it's great not to waste money on a dress that will be worn just once).

If you have younger bridesmaids, too, a colour theme can look great: put little ones in baby blue (or pink), maids of honour in mid-blue (or rosy shade) and the mums in royal blue (or fuchsia). It looks very effective on photographs.

The Final Furlong

Now I have nearly covered every aspect of how to get your look just right, and I hope you're starting to put all your new knowledge into practice. There are just one or two finishing touches left that may need a little attention. So, read on, for the final details.

CHAPTER EIGHT

The Perfect Finish

PUTTING THE ICING ON THE CAKE

large people are easier to spot in a crowd

Wearing clothes that suit you and accessorising well will transform your image, but the effect will be spoiled if your grooming and make-up aren't up to scratch.

Hair Essentials

You will always feel good if your hair is clean and well cared for. Keeping it that way takes time and effort, but the results are worth it. No matter how smart your outfit, how chic your accessories, greasy or untidy hair will always let you down.

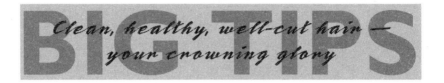

Clean, healthy, well-cut hair — your crowning glory

Beware of sticking to one style for too long — it's too easy to get stuck in a time warp (think of the Queen). It's good to move with the times and have your hair cut in a fashionable style, being careful that it suits you, of course. If you choose a new style from a magazine, consult a professional to have it cut. A professional will always advise you whether your hair and the shape of your head are suitable for the style you like, and if they're not, will suggest a good alternative.

Top hair care tips

- **Always use a pH-balanced shampoo** — if you have dry hair, it won't strip out the natural oils; if you have greasy hair, it won't over-activate the sebaceous glands and make your hair more oily.
- **Always rinse out conditioner thoroughly.** If any is left in, it will make your hair heavy and difficult to manage.
- **Use your hairdryer on a cool or medium setting.** If the air is too hot, it will damage the cuticle of the hair and make it fluffy.
- **Have your hair trimmed regularly** so that you never get caught out by a last-minute invitation.
- If your hair is grey and you colour it, go one or two

shades lighter than your hair used to be — **a darker shade is very ageing.**

- **If your skin is warm toned,** colour with coppery red or golden shades (not cool tones such as ash blonde or ash brown). **If your skin is cool,** try heathery, burgundy or damson shades (not warm tones such as chestnut or gold).
- If you can afford it, **have your hair coloured professionally.**
- **Beware of home perms** — if at all possible, have this done professionally too.
- **Pay attention to the back of your hair** — more people see you from the back than the front.
- Finally, if you do have a slight disaster, it may feel like the end of the world but **it *will* grow out!**

Nails and Hands

Well-groomed hands and nails are as important to your overall appearance as make-up, clean shoes or making sure there isn't a button missing from your blouse. The most pleasant way to ensure your nails always look good is to treat yourself to a weekly manicure.

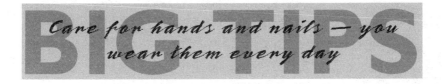

Care for hands and nails — you wear them every day

This can cost as little as £5 or as much as £15 depending on where you live and whether you go to a salon or to a private beautician.

Here are some tips for manicuring your own nails and for looking after your hands and nails between manicures.

- If you don't have the time, money or inclination for a regular manicure or to polish your own nails, **buff them a couple of times a week** so they always have a natural shine and look cared for.
- **Always protect your nails when doing household chores** by wearing cotton gloves for housework and rubber gloves for wet jobs. Water is your nails' worst enemy — it's even more harmful to them than paint stripper!
- As your hands produce very little natural oil and are permanently exposed to wind or sun, the best treatment you can give them is to **moisturise them several times a day.** Keep a jar or tube of your favourite hand cream in your kitchen and bathroom — this will remind you to put moisture back into your hands and nails each time you get them wet. And check that the product you are using contains a sun screen.
- **Look out for acids in nail and hand care products.** With the exception of alphahydroxy, acids dry the nails.
- **Wearing polish will strengthen weak and brittle nails,** but leave it off overnight between polishes to allow air to get to your nails and avoid discoloration.
- **Throw polish away as soon as it begins to thicken** — it lasts longer if you keep it in the fridge.
- The only live part of your nail is the nail-bed, under the cuticle. The only way you can damage your nails

is to damage the nail-bed. **Never cut your cuticles.** If they need attention, here is one of the kindest ways to deal with them:

Cuticle routine

1. In the bath, soak your hands and nails for about ten minutes.
2. Gently push cuticles back with the ball of your thumb — you will probably only need to do this once a week.
3. Dry your nails by slowly using a rotating motion on the cuticle with your towel.
4. Keep some almond oil on your bedside table and massage into your nails and cuticles just before you get into bed.

Manicure

Try this quick and easy manicure routine:

1. Wash your hands thoroughly, scrub nails if necessary.
2. Remove polish — always take polish off with a non-acetone remover. Never pick it off.
3. Clean nails and file them gently with an emery board, not a metal file. File from the edge to the middle in one direction only — not backwards and forwards, as this dries out the nail.
4. Rub hand cream into hands and nails. Remove cream from nails lightly with nail polish remover.
5. Dip nails in water (to remove the remover), dry with a towel.
6. Buff.

You can stop here or continue.

7. Apply one coat of base coat.

8. Apply two coats of your favourite colour.

9. Apply a further top coat.

Emergency repairs

If you wear gloves for chores, a manicure should last you a week. If the polish does chip, though, here's how to effect a quick repair job: brush over the tips of your nails with the same colour as you have on the rest of the nail, allow to dry and re-apply a layer of top coat. Otherwise you need to take off all the polish and start again with a clear coat or a fresh manicure.

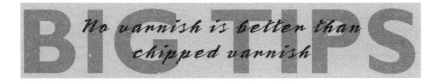

BIG TIPS

No varnish is better than chipped varnish

Note for nail-biters

As you move and speak your hands are instantly noticed. They are your introduction to everyone you meet so, yes, they are a vital part of that first impression, that you mustn't overlook. Bitten nails are unattractive and also imply nervousness or under-confidence.

Nail-biting is a habit which only you have the power to stop. You can try to kick the habit by consulting a hypnotist; or there are products on the market — such as Nail Nurse by Deri — which you paint on to your nails. These have a bitter taste to stop you nibbling and a strengthening agent to help nails grow.

Encouragingly, once you stop biting your nails you will probably end up with much stronger nails than your friends.

Years of nail-biting stimulate your fingers and this produces a strong nail-bed. Does that inspire you? I do hope so.

Skincare

Do you really look after your skin, or do you rely on a hit-and-miss regime? Even if you've never looked after your skin, it's still not too late to start now. You need to cleanse, tone and moisturise your skin morning and evening, whether or not you wear make-up.

I'd like to suggest this easy daily routine which, with a little practice, should only take you a couple of minutes.

I. Cleanse

The first cleanse removes surface dirt and/or make-up.

First take off your eye make-up. Put a little cleanser on some damp cotton wool, wipe eyelashes in a downward and outward movement to remove mascara, turn the cotton wool over and repeat; take a fresh piece of cotton wool and repeat until the cotton wool comes away clean. Once your eye make-up is removed, or if you weren't wearing any, take a piece of damp cotton wool and cleanse the whole eye area, starting in the corner by your nose, using a circular 'C' movement. Repeat on your other eye.

Dot more cleanser around your face and neck and smooth it all over using a gentle upward and outward movement. With the same movement, wipe the cleanser off with damp cotton wool.

This second cleanse removes dirt from pores and dead cells.

Repeat the second cleanse, ideally with a cosmetic sponge (which is very slightly abrasive); or use damp cotton wool again.

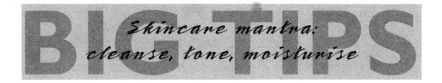

Skincare mantra: cleanse, tone, moisturise

2. Tone

Toning removes any traces of cleanser, helps to refine the pores and to 'perk up' the skin.

Shake a few drops of toner on to some damp cotton wool and gently pat all over your face, starting with your neck and working upwards — avoid your lips and your eye area.

3. Liposome

Liposomes are said to slow down the ageing process and the formation of wrinkles and are usually recommended as soon as facial lines begin to appear (at age thirty or so). Some moisturisers contain liposomes, or these can be used separately as follows.

Use sparingly — dot gently on to any lined areas, such as 'laugh lines' around your eyes, upper lip and forehead. Always include your neck whether you think you need it there or not.

4. Moisturise

Skin loses moisture constantly. Moisturising helps to counteract this process. Some brands are recommended for use morning and evening. Others recommend a different cream for evening use so that in the morning you moisturise and in the evening you nourish your skin.

Dot cream gently around your face and neck and massage in using gentle upward and outward movements, finishing with pressure points on the temple.

On top of your daily routine, I recommend the following on a less frequent basis for really deep-cleansing your skin. Use a masque and/or exfoliator after toning and before moisturising.

1. Mask

Using a mask will give your face a much deeper cleanse than a cleansing cream/lotion. Always use a mask on clean skin. Preferably use an exfoliating cream first (see below) as this will help the mask to penetrate deeper. It is usually recommended that a mask be used once a week for dry skin and two or three times a week for normal to oily skin.

Each brand will have different directions for use. Usually the recommendation is to leave a mask on the skin for a shorter time for dry skin, longer for a normal to oily skin. Read the instructions carefully.

Warning: never use a mask for the first time the night before a big occasion, as it can bring a couple of spots to the surface. This shouldn't happen if you are using a mask on a regular basis.

2. Exfoliate

The top layers of your skin consist of dead cells. Exfoliating regularly removes these dead surface cells, helps to stimulate circulation and should make your skin look younger and fresher. An exfoliator is usually recommended once a week for dry skin and two or three times a week for normal to oily skin.

An exfoliator is slightly abrasive and needs to be massaged gently into the skin, then rinsed off with water or with damp cotton wool.

Cleansing tip

Always work with clean hands and if the creams you use come in pots, never dabble your fingers in them — use a clean spatula instead. (I find tongue depressors, which I order from my local chemist, ideal.) Lotions and potions in dispensers are more hygienic.

Make-up

If you don't generally wear much make-up, bear in mind that research has shown that a well-dressed woman who wears it earns more and is more likely to be promoted than her make-up-free rival — even one with better qualifications.

I find that, on the whole, women who don't wear make-up avoid it because they don't know how to apply it for a natural but professional look. If that's you, then make an appointment for a make-up lesson with your local beautician or image consultant as soon as possible.

If you know you are good with make-up, it's useful to have a quick and easy routine to follow and some hints on how to keep make-up in place all day.

Establish your routine

Always cleanse, tone and moisturise your face and neck before you put on your make-up (always include your neck — this is where the first sign of ageing starts). If you want your make-up to stay in place and look good all day and into the evening too, allow the moisturiser at least five minutes (and preferably, twenty) to sink into your skin before you apply foundation. Do I hear you cry, 'Who has five minutes, let alone twenty, to spare first thing in the morning?' That was my reaction when I was first told about this routine. But it may be that if you change the order in which you get up and get out, you will find that you can make time. For example:

1. Shower.
2. With towel around you cleanse, tone, moisturise.
3. Get dressed.
4. Do your hair.
5. Make the bed.
6. Have a coffee and ...
7. ...make-up.

Practise the following make-up routine until you can easily do it in five minutes (seven minutes absolute maximum).

1. Foundation

Foundation smoothes out any imperfections in your skin and gives a good base for the rest of your make-up. Do buy one that has a sun protection factor. Your foundation should be the same colour as your skin — find the right colour by choosing two or three that look about right (good beauty counters will give you samples) and putting a minute amount of each on a different part of your forehead. Blend into your skin and wait a couple of minutes to see if the pH balance of your skin changes the shade. The best one will be the one that you can't see!

If necessary, use a concealer first on dark shadows under you eyes, or other blemishes. Put a little on to a spatula (not straight on to your skin from a wand as this can spread infection) and apply sparingly. Remove any excess with a dry cosmetic sponge.

Apply foundation all over your face, eyelids and lips with a damp make-up sponge — stop at your jawline, never go below it. Use a light, stippling action — start at the centre of your face and work outwards. (To get the sponge just the right dampness, squeeze it out in a tissue.)

Foundation fact

Unless you have wonderful skin or a sun tan, wearing make-up without foundation is like putting a silk blouse on top of an old, slack bra. Even if your skin *is* good, when you use foundation the make-up will stay in place far longer.

2. Face powder

A loose powder is best, preferably translucent, as this will suit any skin tone, and look good on you when you have a winter pallor as well as when you have a wonderful tan. Powder sets your foundation, helps to absorb any excess moisture and will keep your make-up looking fresh for hours.

Apply with a big brush using light downward strokes — this is important as you have down (small hairs) on your face which you don't want to brush in the wrong direction.

3. Eyebrow pencil

Use this to define, shape and extend your eyebrows if necessary. Eyebrows frame your expression and it is important that they are well defined. If your eyebrows are a good shape but very pale, use a brown or grey eyeshadow instead of a pencil.

Use light, feathery strokes, filling in gaps in your eyebrows.

4. Eyeliner pencil

Your eyes are the windows to your soul — defining them with a pencil will make them look bigger.

Make sure the pencil is sharp. If it is very cold and the pencil feels hard and scratchy, gently warm it between your index finger and thumb.

If you don't usually wear liner, draw a line under one eye only — now examine yourself: the defined eye will look much larger and more interesting.

Unless your eyes are exceptionally large, draw a line under your eyes as close as possible to the eyelashes — a line inside the lower eyelid tends to make your eyes look smaller.

5. Highlighter

Highlighter lightens and brightens your brow bone and acts as a good base for eyeshadow.

Using a brush or a sponge-tipped applicator, apply highlighter all over your eyelid area.

If your eyelids are very wrinkled or you have bulging eyes, use a concealer as a base instead of highlighter.

If you have highly coloured skin pigmentation on your eyelids, use a concealer either before or instead of highlighter.

6. Eyeshadow

This can enhance the colour of your eyes and match or complement the colour of your clothes.

Apply with a brush or eyeshadow applicator.

Always use at least two colours and blend together where they meet.

7. Blusher

Use this to define your cheekbones, highlight your bone structure, add colour to your face and draw attention to your eyes.

Place blusher no lower on your face than in a line with the bottom of your nose.

Always use a large brush (not the little one which is supplied with most compacts) and apply it to your cheekbones with circular movements. Start at your hairline, circle in along your cheek bone and brush back to your hairline.

Apply slightly more than you would like to see as a finished look.

As you finish, *lightly* brush the little blusher which is left on the brush on to your temples — this draws attention to your eyes.

8. Face powder (again)

This second application is to set eyeshadow, highlighter and blusher and will keep them in place for hours.

Apply lightly with brush in a triangle over eyelids and blusher.

Brush lightly backwards and forwards over your cheekbones until your blusher has a 'blended in' look as opposed to an 'I am wearing blusher' look.

9. Mascara

Use to lengthen and thicken your eyelashes.

If you have very straight eyelashes use eyelash curlers before applying mascara.

To coat the wand with mascara, twist it a couple of times in the container. Don't pump the wand up and down — this pushes air into the container, which makes the mascara dry out more quickly.

Apply to your upper lashes first.

Without putting the wand back into the container, apply to your lower lashes — this way there will be just the right amount for a lighter coat on these lower lashes.

10. Lip pencil

Use to shape and define your lips.

Make sure the pencil is sharp. If it is cold and the pencil feels hard, rub it as described for the eyeliner pencil.

Outline your lips, making sure you go right into the corner on your bottom lip as this will give you the illusion of a smile. It also makes an older face look more youthful.

11. Lipstick

A good lipstick will moisturise your lips and protect them from sun and wind as well as enhancing the colour.

For speed, apply from the lipstick itself, inside the lip pencil line.

But for a professional finish which will last for hours:

Apply with a lip-brush inside the lip pencil line.

Blot by taking a tissue, tearing it and separating the sheets so that you have a single layer. Pout, place this single layer of tissue over your lips, brush powder lightly over the tissue, remove tissue and there will be a very fine coat of powder on your lips.

Using a lip-brush, re-apply lipstick and repeat the blotting with a clean tissue — this will give you a matt finish

If you like a shiny finish, re-apply lipstick with a lip-brush.

Tricks or Jokes?

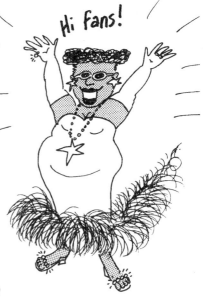

Hi Fans!

There are lots of clever tricks with blushers and highlighters that professionals use to minimise fuller faces, double chins, large noses and so on. But in the hands of the less skilful, you can end up with a full face, double chin or large nose *with stripes*. I'd recommend using the simplest make-up possible. Wear clothes in your best colours and styles, forget the size of your nose and let your personality shine through.

Three-Minute Makeover

When you're pushed for time, skip items 5, 6 and 10 above and apply only one coat of lipstick direct from the stick.

Sweet Smells

Perfume It's lovely to wear it, but keep it discreet for business.

Deodorant Everyone should wear deodorant, whether they think they need it or not. If you know you may have a perspiration problem, wearing natural fibres should help.

The Ultimate Accessory?

Now you're looking wonderful — poised, groomed, elegant and striking — what about your companion? Has the man in your life been intrigued as you've changed your image? Would he like some of the same treatment? Or, perhaps he doesn't think it applies to him, but *you* think you could do with a new-look man to go with your new style? Read the next chapter for a few tips to get him started.

CHAPTER NINE

Men Have Style, Too

HOW TO CREATE THE PERFECT PARTNER
— WE CAN ALL DREAM

ow that you know how to make the most of yourself, can you improve the image of the man in your life? If you're lucky, your man may be intensely interested in this subject; others, like my husband, are born slobs and don't want to know (ever heard someone say, 'You can lead a horse to water, but you can't make it drink'?).

And if you're thinking 'I haven't got a partner', *don't blame it on your size* — go back to Chapter One and read the part called 'Men like big women who like themselves' — it was written with you in mind.

This chapter will help you figure out your partner's style and colour direction. If you shop with him, you will then be able to help him choose wisely. And when it comes to birthday and Christmas presents you'll know just the right things to buy. You may also discover that he's actually been doing you a favour by wearing ties you've chosen for him in the past, and you can let him off the hook!

Whether your partner is a businessman and wears a suit every day or whether he wears mainly casual clothes, *all* men need to know what style of suit is best for them — they'll need to wear one on some occasions. Much of what you have read about yourself relates to your man, too. Let's start as we did with you, by looking at...

His Face Shape

Re-read Chapter Four, pages 80–103 and if he is interested, sit him in front a mirror and work this out together. If he is totally disinterested, don't worry; you can work it out surreptitiously. If he is bald, to work out his face shape you'll have to imagine where his hairline used to be.

Contoured face shape — oval, round, pear or heart
- **Hair** A soft, contoured style will suit his features best.
- **Glasses** Generally speaking a frame which is not too angular is best — refer back to pages 97–103.
- **Ties** Curvy patterns will suit his softened features. Look for Paisleys and curvy foulards (a foulard is a repetitive design or pattern).

Angular face shape — oblong, square, diamond or triangle
- **Hair** An angular style will suit his features best.
- **Glasses** Generally speaking he should go for an angular frame.

- **Ties** Angular patterns will complement his angular features. Look for stripes, angular foulards, pin dots (they form straight lines), polka dots (larger and also forming straight lines, but softer), geometric or abstract patterns.

Body Shapes

Men have just as many different body shapes as women, but for ease I will divide them into three main categories:

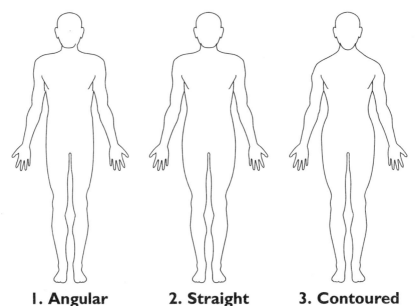

| 1. Angular | 2. Straight | 3. Contoured |

The angular man

- He has very **angular facial features**. (Angular men often have a triangle-shaped face and this is frequently easier to see on a man — if his hair is receding, he can't hide this shape with a fringe.)
- **His shoulders are wider than his hips;** his hips will be noticeably more slender.

The best suit style for this body shape is one cut with a waisted, angular look and quite square shoulders.

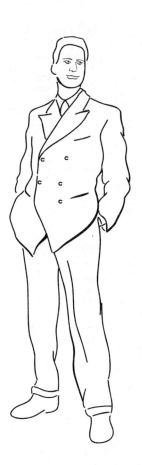

- This is a suit with **an exaggerated line.**
- It can be single- or double-breasted. This style usually has **no vents and looks best with jetted pockets.**
- **A single-breasted suit usually has notched lapels; a double-breasted suit, peaked lapels.**

The overall look your man needs to achieve is crisp, sharp and angular: pin-striped suits; boldly striped shirts; ties with angular patterns.

The straight man
- **His face is probably angular,** but less so than the angular man — often oblong or square, perhaps a softened oblong shape. His face shape could be contoured.
- **His shoulders are in line with his hips** and he often has very little waist.

The best suit style for a straight man is less structured. It still has a straight look — but not a waisted look.

- **This straighter-looking suit comes in single- and double-breasted styles.**
- **It usually has single or double vents and flap pockets.**

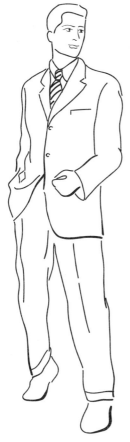

The look is straight and crisp, but not severe.

You are aiming to help him achieve an overall look which is less sharp and angular than the angular man, but still straight and crisp: pin-striped suits with a softer looking stripe, such as a chalk stripe; bird's-eye and herringbone suitings; striped shirts, but less severe than those for an angular man.

If his face is angular, his ties need an angular pattern: stripes, angular foulards, pin dots, geometric or abstract patterns.

If his face is a softened oblong, a certain amount of softness to the pattern of his tie will suit his features: polka dots, for example.

If his face is contoured, softly patterned ties will suit him best: look for ones that feature polka dots, whirly patterns and Paisleys.

The contoured man (guys don't like being called curvy!)
- This man **usually has an oval or round face,** but he may have a straight face shape.
- **If he is slim, he has a defined waistline.**
- **His hips are probably wider than his shoulders.** Or he may have hips in line with his shoulders, but is carrying extra weight and has 'slipped' into this category.

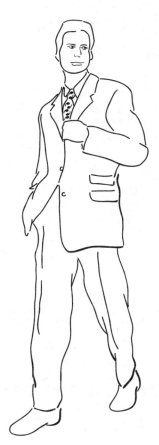

His suits need to have quite a tailored, classic look: a jacket with a very slightly fitted waistline — it needs an ease-of-fit look — and, ideally, flapped pockets. This style usually has a single vent and notched lapels. He needs to achieve an overall softened look to his tailored suits. The cloth can have a self-stripe — pin-stripe is too severe. Bird's-eye, nailhead and plain suitings are excellent choices. Shirts, if striped, should be softly striped. If his face is contoured, he needs ties with curvy patterns. If it's straight, a tie with a more angular pattern will flatter him most.

This is a softer, more contoured look.

Guidelines on Choosing Clothes for Men

Now that you know what shapes and styles will suit him best, here's some more specific, practical advice on choosing men's clothing and ensuring a perfect fit.

Jackets

As fashions come and go, some men stick with what suits them best, others prefer to follow fashion trends. You know your man. I will outline the guidelines but you won't win any Brownie points by trying to get a fashion-conscious man into a double-breasted suit when single-breasted is 'in' (or vice versa).

Double-breasted versus single-breasted

A double-breasted jacket has a broadening and shortening effect and therefore looks best on a slimmer man who is 5ft 7in or taller. Double-breasted looks best on the straight or angular man. It also works well on a slim, contoured man.

A double-breasted jacket should always be worn done up (except when sitting) and the inside button should always be fastened too, to ensure that the jacket hangs correctly.

A single-breasted jacket suits all figure types. It makes a man look taller and slimmer and is therefore the best style for a contoured man or shorter man. If your partner is 6ft 5in and skinny, I would recommend a double-breasted suit.

Whether it's single- or double-breasted, his jacket should fit well at the collar without gaping and he should be able to do it up without the vents pulling across his bottom.

- **Sleeve length** His sleeve should touch his wristbone when he has his arms at his side, and about a quarter of an inch of shirt should show when his arm is bent.
- **Jacket length** Get him to straighten his arm and cup his hand — the bottom of the jacket should just fit into his cupped hand.
- **Buttons** The more formal the jacket, the more buttons on the sleeve — usually four on a dinner jacket or a business suit and two on a casual or sports jacket.
- **Vents** Vents should always lie flat. Be careful if he is broad in the beam — two vents can have a widening effect.

Trousers

He should be able to insert two fingers widthways into the waistband. If not, his trousers are too tight.

- **Pockets** should lie flat — if they flare out, he needs a larger size.
- **Pleats** should drape and hang easily — again, if they flare, he needs a larger size, or a different style.
- **Belt v. braces** If he is a large man or has a beer gut, braces will often make his trousers hang much better than a belt. And they'll hang even better if the waist is one inch too big. If the trousers have belt hoops then a belt should always be worn. If he wears braces, the belt hoops must be removed — it's one or the other, not both!

- **Turn-ups** make legs look shorter and general advice
  is that he needs to be over 5ft 7in to wear them. But
  if he has no problem about being short and likes
  turn-ups — fine!
- **Trouser bottoms** should touch the middle of the
  back of the shoe and should be half an inch shorter
  in front.

Trouser tip

Before having trousers shortened get him to transfer
everything he usually carries around with him (keys, loose
change etc.) into the pockets. They can make the trousers as
much as an inch longer!

Suits

Whenever possible, he should buy two pairs of trousers to a
suit and alternate them to ensure that each pair has equal
wear. For the same reason, all three pieces should be dry
cleaned at the same time.

- If he wears a suit daily, **he needs at least three
  suits,** preferably five plus. His suits will last longer if
  he wears them in rotation.
- **When suit shopping, make sure he wears a
  shirt, tie and business shoes.** You really can't tell
  if the suit's right if he's wearing a sweatshirt, no tie
  and gym shoes!

Shirts

His shirt collar should show above his jacket collar at the
front and the back.

- **Collar size** Check it for him every six months by measuring around his neck under his Adam's apple. Many men keep on wearing the same collar size as they wore at school! A good fit is snug — neither too tight nor too loose.
- **Collar shape** If he has a long neck, a high-cut collar is best. Short collars make a long neck look longer. Likewise, if he has a short neck, a lower-cut one is best. Long collars make a short neck look longer.

Ties

These are important. They should always finish at the trouser waistband. If it finishes above, he'll look like a schoolboy. If it finishes below, he'll look out of proportion. The better quality the tie, the better he'll look.

Socks

- **When he is sitting with crossed legs you shouldn't be able to see any skin.** Tell him most women find it a complete turn off to see an expanse of hairy leg!
- **His socks should be the same colour as either his shoes or his trousers.** White socks are banned with a business suit. Plain socks are more appropriate than patterned.

Shoes

As with suits, it is preferable not to wear the same pair of shoes daily, so he should have *at least* two pairs to alternate.

- **Shoes should always be the same colour as, or darker than, his trousers.**
- **See advice on pages 62–3 as regards shoe care:** shoetrees, polish, driving, etc.

Glasses

- **If he can't be bothered to clean his glasses regularly, do it for him.** Nothing is worse than looking at a man's eyes through a veil of dust.

Other accessories

Watch and other jewellery, briefcase, wallet, belt, etc. need to be the best quality he can afford because they convey so many unspoken messages about his status.

Grooming for Men

Hair

- **Balding men** may need to be advised to stop parting their hair and combing the strands across the bald part, and encouraged to brush it straight back instead.
- **The hair care tips on page 156 apply just as much to your man as to you.**
- **A clean-shaven look is often said to be more professional,** but if he is a successful, professional man with a beard and he likes himself that way — *shush!*
- **Beards and moustaches or designer stubble are best confined to the 'media' man.**

General grooming

- **Nothing can beat a good hairstyle and a clean, neat appearance.**
- **Encourage him to make sure his nails are always clean and filed.** Treat him to an occasional manicure, he'll be amazed at the difference it makes to his hands. If he thinks it's not 'macho', 'sell' it to him by telling him it's an extremely relaxing and de-stressing experience.
- **To ensure that his trousers always look immaculate, invest in a trouser press** (you'll probably use it as often as he does once he's bought it).
- **Everyone should wear a deodorant, whether they need one or not.**
- **After-shave should be discreet for business.**
- **Men with a strong beard should keep a razor at work** — there's nothing worse than a five o'clock shadow at an evening meeting.
- Although many men wince at the idea, **skin care is just as important for men as for women.** There are lots of unperfumed lotions around that you could share — and, increasingly, there are excellent products for men on the market.

Colour for Men

As with women, there are many dress code 'rules' for men. Some men like to adhere to them strictly, others prefer to use them as guidelines rather than tramlines.

The city suit

In the corporate world men tend to have a 'uniform', the City look — dark navy suits (or sometimes dark grey), white shirts and, often, indifferent ties. They know this can be boring and would often like to look more exciting, but have been a bit unsure how to go about it and are scared to try in case they don't achieve the desired effect.

Men in more artistic professions — the media, advertising, etc.— will more happily wear suits in lighter, more interesting tones and some will try unusual, contemporary colour combinations.

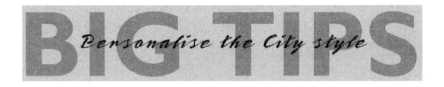

BIG TIPS *Personalise the City style*

The classic City style gives the professional man a universally recognised look that conveys honesty, authority and professionalism. If, when you read about colour, you can see that light navy is better than dark navy for him, he won't listen to you anyway. So a City-type man, whether he is warm or cool, light or deep, bright or muted, needs to be shown how to wear that dark navy suit. He can use his shirt and tie to make his 'uniform' work for him as an individual.

Warm or cool test for men

Look back at Chapter Six, particularly page 131. Is your man predominantly warm or cool? If he finds this subject interesting, you can look together at the colours of his favourite sweaters, ties and T-shirts; if not, you'll either have to observe or casually ask him about these.

1. Look at his ties. Group together the ones he wears most
   — that's usually between 4 and 10. Look at the background
   colours. What dark shades does he seem to prefer?
   a) Navy; a strong, rich burgundy; charcoal grey.
   b) Dark teal (a deep, greeny blue); a brown burgundy;
      deep rust.
2. What colours are the patterns? Are they mainly:
   a) blue reds; red burgundies; blue greens?
   b) peachy tones; orange reds; yellowy greens?
3. Does he prefer himself/look best in:
   a) a white or soft white shirt?
   b) an ivory or a cream shirt?
4. In the sun, wearing a low-factor lotion, does he:
   a) burn easily?
   b) tan gradually?
5. For a casual sweater, track suit or T-shirt, does he
   prefer/look best in:
   a) blues; blue reds; navy; black?
   b) browns; rusts; oranges; teals?
6. If he likes striped shirts, does he buy stripes which are
   mainly:
   a) blue reds; blue greens; pinks?
   b) browns; peaches; oranges?

Rating:

If he scored four or more (a)s, he looks best in *cool* tones.
If he scored four or more (b)s, he looks best in *warm* tones.

Bright or muted?

1. Look in his wardrobe. Are most of his casual clothes:
   a) brightly coloured?
   b) or do they have a soft quality to the colours?

2. Look at his ties. Are the ones he favours:
   a) brightly coloured?
   b) or do they have a more blended, quieter look?

Rating:
If the answers were both (a), he likes contrast in the clothes that he wears — he looks best in vibrant colours and his colour direction is bright.

If the answers were both (b) and most of his clothes have a soft, hazy look about them, he looks best in soft tones and his colour direction is muted.

Deep or light?
Think about him in a polo or crew-necked sweater. Which would look better on him — a deep shade or a light colour? Whichever looks best tells you whether his direction is deep or light.

By now you should be able to assess whether he looks best in bright or soft; deep or light; cool tones (Winter/Summer) or warm tones (Autumn/Spring).

The warm/cool double-check
Imagine him wearing a dark navy blazer with a white shirt. Tick which groups of colours in a tie would make his face come to life:

a) Bright, high-contrast colours — a clear, bright red; an emerald green; bright, clear blue.
b) Bright, but lighter, tones — an orangey red; a lime green; peach.
c) Truly warm colours — orange; orange red; bright gold; coral.

d) Intensely cool, blue-toned colours, but not as bright as (a) — blue reds; blue greens; a soft, deep blue.

e) Light, soft, pastel shades — baby blue; light, pale blue green; silver grey.

f) Light but warm colours — light, peachy tones; light, yellowy green; light aquas.

g) Muted softened tones, which have a 'dusty' quality about them — a soft medley of pinks, blues, pale greys, greens.

h) Soft, monochrome colours — such as blends of beige, browns and rusts; soft golds and mustards; or soft peachy tones and camels.

i) Deep, warm, intense colours — rusts; deep orange; dark, olive green.

j) Deep, cool, bold colours — burgundies; pine green; royal blue; charcoal grey.

Rating:

If your answer to the warm/cool quiz was *warm,* you probably ticked some of the following: b, c, f, h, i (Autumn/Spring).

If your answer to the warm/cool quiz was *cool,* you probably ticked some of the following: a, d, e, g, j (Winter/Summer).

Finer Colour Points

I hope you are beginning to picture the best colours for your partner to wear for his ties and for casual wear (the colours he wears by his face).

By now you will probably have decided whether he is a 'cool' or a 'warm' person. I hope you have also managed to decide whether his colour direction is 'bright' or 'muted', 'light' or 'deep'. Now on to some of the finer points on colour.

With a suit or blazer, his ties need to reflect his colour direction. When he is dressed casually, then his sweaters, T-shirts, track suits will look best on him in these tones too.

- If he is **bright**, he needs to wear bright colours by his face — jewel colours; bright, clear red; blue; green.
- If he is **muted**, he should go for softened, hazy tones by his face — soft, warm blends of peaches, rusts and creams (warm); or soft, cool blends of blues, smoky greys, pinks and greens (cool).
- If he is **warm**, he needs to wear golden tones by his face — orange; mustard; lime green; or teal.
- If he is **cool**, he should try cool tones by his face — magenta; cerise; emerald green; or cherry red.
- If he is **light**, he needs light tones by his face — cool, powdery blues, greens and pinks; or warm, light tones of peach and yellowy greens.
- If he is **deep**, he'll look best with deep tones by his face — dark navy; pine green; deep burgundy; royal blue (cool); or warm, deep tones of rusts, browns, forest green (warm).

White versus cream
- If he is **warm,** his best 'white' will be either ivory, oyster or cream. These will enhance his skin tone, while white will always look clinical on him.
- If he is **cool,** clear white or a soft white is best for him. These will clarify his skin and make it look

vibrant and alive while cream or ivory will deaden it and may make him look sallow. If he is clean-shaven, ivory and, particularly, cream can make him look as if he hasn't shaved properly.

Gold versus silver

- If you have decided that your man is a *warm* person, gold will look better than silver for any of his accessories.
- If you have decided he is a *cool* person, silver will look better against his skin-tone than gold — remember this when you buy him a watch, a ring or a pen, or help him to choose new glasses.

The Way Forward

I hope that by giving your partner the once-over you have accurately assessed his style and his colours but, just as for yourself, the only way to be *really* sure you've got it right is for him to have a professional analysis — go on, see if you can talk him into it.

Epilogue

OVER TO YOU…

'NOBODY WILL PUT ON YOUR TOMBSTONE
WHETHER YOU HAD BLACK COFFEE,
COFFEE WITH CREAM OR BLACK FOREST GATEAU,
NOR HOW MUCH YOU WEIGHED.
YOU ONLY GET ONE CRACK AT LIFE
— NO REHEARSALS, NO ENCORES. ENJOY IT.
AND IF THAT MEANS ENJOYING
WHAT YOU EAT, DO IT.'

John Neville — Plus Sizes Fashion Designer

I hope that you have found *Big Living* inspiring and helpful, and that you'll try out at least some of my suggestions. They are all designed to make you feel at ease with the size you are today and to develop your style around it. If you take a good look at yourself and evaluate honestly who you are and how you come across to others, you will see where you can improve. Just remember always to be true to the real you — you don't want to change *who* you are, you want to make the most of yourself.

I've tried to help you identify what really suits you — your shape, your colouring and, of course, your personality. Knowing exactly what you want and need will save you time and money when you go shopping. Enjoy buying clothes for the shape you are and don't be restricted to wearing just one or two outfits. Aim to have a wardrobe full of clothes that fit and mix and match, too. Your final aim is to be able to look in the mirror and smile because you like what you see.

This dream wardrobe won't happen overnight. But, following my guidelines, it will happen gradually, and within your own budget. As it grows and develops, so will your confidence in yourself and the way you look. When you have that confidence, you project a positive image and people respond to it. This time next year, do the two quizzes in Chapter One again. I'm sure you'll notice the difference in your perception of yourself — and you'll probably already have noticed the difference in the way people behave towards you.

Now it's up to you. Go out there and live life to the full.

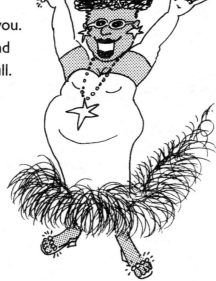

Bibliography

Diet Breaking: Mary Evans Young: Published by Hodder and Stoughton

You Count, Calories Don't: Linda Omichinski R.D. with Mary Evans Young: Published by Hodder and Stoughton

The Forbidden Body — Why Being Fat is not a Sin: Shelley Bovey: Published by Pandora Press

Yes!: Leading bi-monthly magazine with a positive approach to life, health and fashion for the size 16+ woman: Editor Janice Bhend. Available at major newsagents.

Executive Woman: Monthly magazine for the business woman: editor Angela Giveon. Available at newsagents or by subscription.

Useful Information

Corporate and private Image Consultancy services
Angela Sandler AMFIC
'The Studio', 13 Glanleam Road, Stanmore, Middx. HA7 4NW
Tel and Fax: 0181 954 2113

Training courses in Image Consultancy
Suzi Pickles AMFIC
The Colour Company, Quince Cottage, 126 Tonbridge Road, Hildenborough, Kent TN11 9EN
Tel and Fax: 01732 833 334

The Federation of Image Consultants
President: Penny Scott Blackhall AMFIC 01455 845 436
Membership Secretary: Jennifer Gauld AMFIC 01732 867 492
Consultant in your local area: Jean Parkes 0956 701 018